'Beyrer writes with the rigour of an outstanding scientist, and the compassion and energy of a tireless advocate.'

Peter Piot, Director of the London School of
Hygiene & Tropical Medicine

'Beyrer has an almost encyclopaedic knowledge of the global HIV epidemic that this book so richly describes. More than any other Western researcher, he understands the cultural and political factors that impact local epidemics.'

Adeeba Kamarulzaman, Dean of the University of
Malaya Faculty of Medicine

'Offers honest insights on sex between men, drug use, sex work, and transgender people in Southeast Asia. Chris Beyrer offers pragmatic solutions to inspire a new generation of leaders.'

Midnight Poonkasetwattana, Asia-Pacific Community of
MSM Organizations (APCOM)

About the author

Chris Beyrer is the Desmond Tutu professor in
public health and human rights at Johns Hopkins
University, and was formerly president of the
International AIDS Society. He has extensive
experience in conducting international research
and training programs on HIV/AIDS around
the world, and has served as an advisor on HIV
prevention to international bodies including
the World Bank, the United States Office of
AIDS Research, and the Thai Red Cross. His
other published works include the edited
collection *Public Health and Human Rights:
Evidence-Based Approaches* (2007).

WAR IN THE BLOOD

SEX, POLITICS AND AIDS IN SOUTHEAST ASIA

Second edition

Chris Beyrer

ZED
Zed Books
London

War in the Blood: Sex, Politics and AIDS in Southeast Asia was
first published in 1997 by Zed Books Ltd, The Foundry,
17 Oval Way, London SE11 5RR, UK.

This edition was published in 2017

www.zedbooks.net

Typeset in Plantin and Kievit by Swales & Willis Ltd, Exeter, Devon
Index by ed.emery@thefreeuniversity.net
Cover design by Clare Turner

A catalogue record for this book is available from the British Library.

ISBN 978-1-78699-194-2 hb
ISBN 978-1-78699-193-5 pb
ISBN 978-1-78699-195-9 pdf
ISBN 978-1-78699-196-6 epub
ISBN 978-1-78699-197-3 mobi

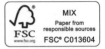

MIX
Paper from
responsible sources
FSC® C013604
www.fsc.org

Printed by CPI Group (UK) Ltd, Croydon, CR0 4YY

CONTENTS

PREFACE TO THE SECOND EDITION

Imagine an end to AIDS.

We may now have the tools in hand to conquer this virus. We even have a target in sight – the end of AIDS as a public health threat by 2030, put forward by the UN and widely embraced. It is not at all certain that we will achieve control of the greatest infectious disease epidemic of our time, already the killer of 40 million people. But with a renewed push, with universal access to treatment and the skillful use of new prevention tools, we might just break the back of AIDS. The very idea was unimaginable in the 1990s when I lived and worked in Southeast Asia – the period of explosive spread of the virus among the peoples of the region.

War in the Blood was written in 1996–1997, and published in 1997. It was my first book. To my surprise and admitted delight it has stayed in print and continued to be read and used despite great changes in the HIV pandemic – and the markedly altered political and social landscapes of Southeast Asia. But AIDS, the world, and your author have changed. It was past time for an update.

In 1996, effective treatment for HIV infection and clinical AIDS had come at last. For those fortunate women, men, and children living with the virus in the wealthiest countries, the dying of the 1980s and 1990s had abruptly stopped. We called this the Lazarus effect, after the biblical figure Christ raised from the dead. And in New York and San Francisco, London and Paris, Sydney and Amsterdam, desperately ill people truly did rise up from their beds, regain lost weight, recover resistance, live. The early regimens were complex and costly, some side effects brutal, and not everyone got on therapy in time to be saved. But this was a true watershed. The end of the death sentence.

For the peoples of Southeast Asia, indeed for the more than 90 percent of people living with the virus worldwide, the Lazarus effect of 1996 was a tantalizing rumor. Not only had treatment not become available for all but the wealthiest few – it was barely being considered. Drug costs, then at around $22,000 per year, were prohibitive.

Treatment regimens and the clinical management of AIDS patients was thought too complex for many fragile health systems. The foci of virtually all programs in the region remained on prevention, on stigma reduction, management of opportunistic infections, and, for those in the last stages of AIDS, palliative care. In re-reading and re-thinking this book, the most striking change from then till now is that the period the book covered was before the world committed to treatment in developing countries. The late 1990s were a searing interregnum when we had treatment and most with HIV had no hope of getting it. In 2016, as I write, we have marked an extraordinary milestone, not just in global health but in human solidarity, with 17 million people worldwide on treatment. And amazingly, most of those millions live in the most heavily burdened countries of the world – South Africa, Kenya, Botswana, India, Thailand. The world truly did rally to the AIDS crisis.

The scale and scope of the AIDS treatment rollout was unprecedented, though it took a decade after the development of therapy before substantial numbers of lives would be saved. Treatment access began in earnest in 2003, seven years after triple therapy had been found effective, with the establishment of two landmark programs: UN Secretary-General Kofi Annan's Global Fund to Fight AIDS, TB and Malaria (GFATM), and U.S. President George W. Bush's signature President's Emergency Fund for AIDS Relief (PEPFAR). PEPFAR began as a $15 billion, five-year commitment on the part of the Bush administration. It was primarily focused on Africa, with Haiti and Guyana in the Americas included, and just one country in Asia, Vietnam. PEPFAR had been memorably announced during the president's 2003 State of the Union address. It came as a shock to many, including my partner (now husband) Mike and I, who watched that address, anxious to hear as were so many, what the President would say regarding the impending disaster of the Iraq invasion. We weren't sure we'd heard the short statement on AIDS correctly. Really? Fifteen billion dollars for global AIDS? Yes, as it turned out. A commitment which the Bush administration met, then exceeded, and which President Obama continued and expanded.

HIV treatment is now so simple, often a single tablet once a day, and so effective, that the term 'AIDS' itself has a somewhat dated ring. Leaders in the field have questioned whether we should still be using it – suggesting 'HIV disease' as a better capture of the clinical spectrum we're now working with – where most people with the virus need never develop AIDS. Where treatment is available this has become an outpatient disease.

Later work would reveal an additional and transformative benefit to HIV treatment. Successful control of the virus in the body's tissues and fluids, of viremia, renders those treated dramatically less infectious. This is true in sex, in pregnancy, and in breast feeding. Treatment is prevention. But the drugs only work if you take them. Inconsistent or episodic use can lead to the emergence of drug resistance and treatment failure. This can be an individual issue, say with someone with a chaotic life – or it can be a problem of weak or dysfunctional health systems. Russia, to name one hard case, has been plagued by drug stock outs and shortages in her federal HIV treatment centers, challenging even the most committed patients and their providers.

How else has HIV changed? The research agenda has dramatically expanded – and now includes an intense effort around a cure. One man, Timothy Brown, known as the Berlin Patient, has been demonstrably cured of HIV infection,[1] several cases of long-term remission off therapy have been described, and young scientists worldwide have taken on HIV cure research as the next great scientific challenge in the field.

Research advances have also transformed the prevention landscape. First and foremost, the insight that effective treatment has such potent prevention benefits. Second is the impressive benefit of male circumcision on reducing a man's risk of acquiring HIV from an infected woman. Three trials, all done among African men, showed consistent HIV risk reductions of about 60 percent for circumcision. The lack of male circumcision among the predominately Buddhist populations of Burma, Thailand, and Cambodia is now understood to have contributed to the rapid heterosexual epidemics which occurred in all three countries. The converse was true for Muslim majority Malaysia, and for the Philippines, where traditional male circumcision is ubiquitous and pre-dates the Catholicism of the archipelago – and where rates in heterosexual men (those who didn't inject drugs) stayed low.

After many failed attempts, one HIV vaccine trial, conducted by the U.S. military HIV research program with the Thai Ministry of Public Health (the program described in Part Two of this book),

RV144, has shown modest, transient efficacy, signaling possible ways forward for a vaccine.

And perhaps most importantly, a potent new prevention tool, pre-exposure prophylaxis, or PrEP, has shown remarkable ability to protect against HIV infection. PrEP is the use of an oral antiviral drug, more commonly of the two drug combination Truvada,[2] for HIV uninfected persons at risk. PrEP has shown consistent effectiveness for gay men, for the uninfected male and female partners of people living with the virus, in one trial for people who inject drugs. It works. It could have made a world of difference to my late partner, Ed and I, but was decades in the future when he was so ill and our prevention options so few.

In sum, HIV in 2016 is a strikingly different epidemic than the one described in this book in 1998.

Yet too many aspects of the pandemic, of our responses to it, have not changed. Or not changed enough to achieve epidemic control. Fewer than half of the estimated 38.8 million people living with HIV worldwide are on treatment. Health disparities for the poor in the global North, including in the U.S., remain too wide for conscience or control. And most importantly, new HIV infections, incident infections, among adults are stable in much of the world and rising in at least two regions,[3] insuring that the pandemic continues to expand. New infections have held stubbornly steady since 2010 across Southeast Asia as well. Some of this is due to good news – the longer survival of people with HIV on effective treatment. But much of it is due to something more troubling, and at the heart of *War in the Blood* – the failure to reach and to protect those most burdened – gay men, sex workers, people who inject drugs, transgender women, and adolescent girls and young women whose only real risk is starting sexual life. We didn't have a term for these diverse communities in 1998. We first referred to them as Most at Risk Populations. Now they are grouped as Key Populations. Whatever the term, the harsh truth is that we were failing them in the 1990s, and largely, we still are.

The reasons for these failures now, as then, are not related simply to funding, or the challenges of changing behaviors. What remains true and truly bedeviling is that governments, communities, families – our own hearts and minds – continue to struggle with the realities of sex, with sexuality and with gender, with drug use and drug dependency. It remains stubbornly the case that our inability to adopt pragmatic and humane public health approaches continues to aid and abet the virus, not those we seek to protect.

Southeast Asia has done well in responding to HIV and AIDS on many fronts. Thailand was the first Asian country to implement universal access to antiretroviral therapy (ART), and the first, in 2016, to be certified free of mother-to-child transmission of HIV by the World Health Organization. Cambodia achieved remarkable success in controlling heterosexual spread, despite her continued poverty and weak health system. Yet an explosive epidemic of HIV continues among the region's young gay men and among her transgender women – and rates remain high in sex workers of all three genders.

Wars in the blood continue in the region. And that is why it seemed worth updating this book. I sincerely wish it were now primarily of historical interest. But that, tragically, is not the case.

Et moi? I arrived in Chiang Mai, northern Thailand, in 1992 to start work as the field director for a new collaborative project on HIV research between Johns Hopkins University and Chiang Mai University. I was 33, alone, and in deep grief over the recent death of my first lover from pulmonary Kaposi's Sarcoma, an AIDS-related cancer. That fall I had finished my training at Johns Hopkins and was unsure what to do next. I knew only that I had to leave New York, where I was from and where my partner and so many of our circle had died. Thailand saved my life. I mean that literally. Starting a new job, building a new circle of friends, eventually starting to see men again. Being in a deep Buddhist culture where practice was made easier, simpler, by the piety of my Thai friends, by the alluring beauty of Chiang Mai's many temples, and by the subtle and clarifying tradition of vipassana, insight meditation.

Chiang Mai and her Buddhist culture are a renowned center for the teaching and practice of vipassana, a simple but deep practice focused on mindfulness. It has no prayers, no mantras, no visualizations. Instead the focus is all on mindful attention to the breath, the body, and the state of consciousness. On paying attention to the flow of the mind to gain insight, clearing consciousness of its distracting clutter, noise, and confusion. It is, some scholars argue, as close to the original teachings of the historical Buddha as one can get. I hadn't known this when I arrived. It was the Thai nurses at the university, serious practitioners, who brought me to several renowned insight meditation teachers, gave me books on the practice, and arranged for weekend retreats where I could learn in earnest.

It took two years of hard grieving to recover from Ed's loss. Eventually, though, I did – or thought I had. What followed was a period of intense sexual desire, more intense than anything I'd known. Chiang Mai was a good place for connecting with men, Thais and other expats, and then there was also Bangkok with its huge scene, and KL, smaller but more sophisticated. It was a heady time. What was less fabulous, and which gradually became terrifying, was that mixed in with my desire for men was something new. A desire for unsafe sex.

For the Buddha's teaching that there is a remedy for craving, for attachment, and that that remedy is inside ourselves and can be reached through meditation, I know I owe my life. Rather than give up condoms (or men) I went into a vipassana retreat at a meditation center in the forests outside of Chiang Mai. This was to be a week-long retreat following the Thai monastic regimen. Lay people were to wear only white, abstain from alcohol, meat, drugs, sex. Two meals a day were served, a predawn breakfast and a lunch before noon, after that, only water or tea. There was sweeping up the compound, a daily meeting with a meditation teacher, and otherwise, nothing but practice, practice, practice.

What followed was one of the most painful experiences I've endured. It was literally excruciating to sit, stand, walk, in mindfulness practice for hours a day, digging into the grief, the layered losses. Opening into terrible wells of loneliness. Sadnesses I hadn't known were there. It got steadily worse each day, leading to afternoon migraines of throbbing intensity. But after several days I did get to the insight part of the practice. On about the fifth day I finally realized that what was driving me was love. Not love for life or for the living. It was love, identification, with the men I'd lost. With Ed. I didn't want to survive – I wanted, so deeply, to be with the dead and not the living. With that insight, slowly, the practice got better. My guide, a grave young Spaniard who was deciding whether to ordain as a monk, noticed this on the next to last day of the retreat. He said simply 'I see you've dropped something. You're lighter today.' And I was.

Remarkably enough, when I slipped back into ordinary life, the desire to engage in risk was gone. It never returned.

I stayed in Thailand for five years. During those years I taught, ran studies, and traveled the AIDS road in Thailand, Burma, Laos, Cambodia, Vietnam, Malaysia, and China. In 1997 I returned to the U.S. to take up a new position as head of Johns Hopkins Fogarty AIDS International Training and Research Program. That work included supporting training and research with our partners in Southeast Asia, but also grew to include India, and Russia. Most challenging for me, the program had a large number of ongoing projects in Africa. In Ethiopia, Malawi, South Africa, and Uganda, where Hopkins researchers had been engaged in the devastating African epidemics of HIV and TB. Working on AIDS in Asia didn't prepare me for the scale and scope of the African epidemics – perhaps nothing could. Ancient, deeply impoverished Ethiopia was the first country we took on. Working there made me appreciate the relative ease, the wealth, of a Thailand or a Malaysia. How much we'd had to work with. And to feel the enormity of the wave of suffering and dying that Africans were facing.

I kept working on HIV and on health and human rights projects in Thailand, China, and Laos. In Burma, I was banned for 11 years after doing a training for the NLD youth on HIV – but continued to work on multiple projects from across the Thai–Burma and India–Burma borders. I became a professor, and then the Desmond Tutu Professor in Public Health and Human Rights at Johns Hopkins. Like many of my peers and friends doing this work, I gradually became a commuter – no longer the young guy fulltime in the field. Travel to Southeast Asia was one or two times a year, sometimes three, as work pulled me more widely across the AIDS road. That road led to Central Asia – Tajikistan and Kazakhstan – as HIV spread among drug users in the Golden Crescent lands, and to more than a decade of work in the Russian Federation herself – tough slogs with sex workers and gay men in an increasingly repressive state.

In 2014, I was elected President of the International AIDS Society, the largest professional body in our field.

With the defeat of the Defense of Marriage Act in 2013, I became something else – a legally married man, and at 53, a citizen with full rights for the first time in my life. It's hard for those who have lived with unquestioned rights, like marriage, inheritance, adoption – just plain social acceptance – to understand how powerful gaining such basic rights can be.

In 2016 it looks as though Taiwan may break the current Asian log jam on marriage equality. It is a consummation devoutly to be wished.

★ ★ ★

My debts and thanks to the many friends and colleagues acknowledged in the first edition of this book continue. The dedication to my friend Peter Lange must now be In Memoriam since Peter passed away, just as I began work on this edition, in his home of Chiang Mai in October of 2016. Peter had served as the administrator of the Johns Hopkins–Chiang Mai University program for the years 1992–1997 when I too was fortunate to live and work in that lovely old city. One of the few foreigners to achieve the status of *karatchakan*, a civil servant of the Royal Thai Government, Peter shared unstintingly his deep knowledge and love of all things Thai – and kept an eager young American from making countless mistakes.

Our wonderful group at the Center for Public Health and Human Rights at Johns Hopkins have been invaluable in our ongoing work in Southeast Asia, and in allowing me the time to work on this revision. Deep thanks to Stef Baral, Andrea Wirtz, Emily Clouse, Michele Decker, Brian Weir, Sandra Mon, Vit Suwanvanichkij, and Nick Thomson.

My husband, Michael Smit, makes this work possible and life itself joyous.

I must add an additional deep thanks to the Rockefeller Foundation for their generosity in offering me a residency at their retreat center in resplendent Bellagio, Italy to revise this book. Time is the only real luxury.

INTRODUCTION

We were walking down a street in the seaside resort city of Pattaya, just south of ceaselessly expanding Bangkok. January, 2016 – even in this coolest season a sweaty stroll. My companions were two friends from SWING, Khun Surang, a petite dynamo of a woman who heads up the group, and her second in command, Khun Tee, a bawdy fellow who knew all the owners and managers of the venues we were visiting – and whose teasing and good humor were our ticket into the scene. SWING, the Sex Workers in Union Group, is a Thai union for sex workers. Its members include women, men, and transfolk who sell sex in the still enormous Thai industry. They were our partners for a new project working to bring pre-exposure prophylaxis, PrEP, to men selling sex, since it was clear to SWING and to us that conventional HIV prevention was failing these young men. We'd already agreed to work together on providing PrEP at SWING's clinic in the red light district of Silom, in Bangkok's entertainment zone, one of the world's largest (Bangkok had 68 gay sex venues enumerated by SWING in 2016 – with an estimated 36,000 workers). But it was at Khun Surang's insistence that we were in Pattaya together. She wanted me to meet the men from Cambodia.

Pattaya has many zones. The straight venues focus on bar girls, topless shows, outright brothels. They cater to a diverse clientele – the signs are the giveaways – in Chinese, Korean, Cyrillic for the Russians, and of course, Thai. There is a vibrant *katoey*, or transgender scene. The clubs and cabarets here are famous for Las Vegas-style showgirl extravaganzas, featuring lip synching to the latest pop, lots of feathers, long legs, big hair, and strikingly pretty female faces (all born male, to be clear). Sisters, the transwomen's advocacy group, whom we met on our next trip to Pattaya, estimates that 75 percent of the transgender women in town sell sex. They do this to survive and to send money to families back home in the provinces, as dutiful Thai daughters are culturally bound to do. Then there is Boyz Town, the big bustling gay district that caters to Thais and foreigners alike, and where the young Thai men working in the bars and clubs are known for being both handsome and accommodating. This is the high end of Pattaya's trade. At the low end are the Khmers.

While the Thai economy has stalled in the past decade of political turmoil and military rule, the double digit growth of the 1990s now past, it remains a substantially larger and more robust economy than those of Thailand's still impoverished neighbors, Burma, Laos, and Cambodia. In 1998 Hun Sen was consolidating power in Cambodia and looking very much like what he has subsequently become – a dictator determined to thwart all rivals. He has been continuously in power ever since. Cambodia's political, social, and economic life has stalled under his authoritarian and corrupt rule. This has made labor migration to Thailand one of few opportunities open to many impoverished Khmers. Including LGBT ones.

Khun Surang and Khun Tee had asked us to come to this particular street in Pattaya because they were hoping we'd consider including migrant sex workers in our PrEP program. What greeted us that sweaty afternoon was a long string of bars, restaurants, and clubs, tightly packed along both sides of a winding sun-blasted street. We counted over 30 venues just in eyesight. It was a late Sunday afternoon, before happy hour, and the men were dressed and pressed for the evening ahead. To a one, every worker we met was from Cambodia. Most were openly gay, some blending gender roles, with heavy makeup or long hair, painted nails. A distressingly large number had the obvious muscle wasting and skin lesions of advanced HIV disease, one a burning vesicular lesion of oral herpes which he'd treated with gentian violet, an over-the-counter tincture that had stained half his lower face purple. They were a hungry-looking group. The clientele at this early hour were an older crowd – mostly men over 60 – some much older. My SWING friends said that this area was more popular with foreign retirees then with tourists or locals. Drinks were cheaper than in Boyz Town and the vibe much more relaxed.

How about HIV infection rates among these men? They were selling sex in a country with high rates of HIV testing, a policy of universal access to ART (for Thai citizens and registered migrant workers at least), and which had just been declared free of mother-to-child transmission of HIV. We don't have data broken out by ethnicity or nationality – but we do know that young men who have sex with men (MSM) have higher rates of new infection now than any other group in Thailand. Some 5–12 percent are becoming newly infected each year, with the highest rates, over 8 percent per year, among the youngest men, aged 18–21, and among the subset who sell sex. This is an explosive epidemic and a sustained one. And it appears to be dislinked from heterosexual spread, which in Thailand, as in Cambodia, has come under remarkable control.

Who would have predicted that the future of AIDS would look so much like the past – with the most affected people again being young gay men?

Thailand *is* by many measures a success story in AIDS. But the epidemic affecting her young gay men is part of a wider trend underway not just in the country, or the region, but globally – a new wave of HIV infections among young gay men despite all the successes of the past three decades.

Understanding HIV in the region now requires that we interrogate the current programs and policies of these diverse states, and do so in the light of the tremendous scientific and clinical advances of the past decades. It also requires that we think about the largely stalled hopes for development, democracy, and human rights – fronts on which the states of mainland Southeast Asia have struggled to make headway – and on which many have abjectly failed. Thailand illustrates all too many of these failures.

In the 1990s political thinkers, my Thai colleagues and friends, spoke confidently about the end of the cycle of weak civilian regimes upended by military coups. In retrospect, what looked like a nascent, but ever-firmer basis in democracy in the 1990s, was actually the high water mark for the Thai political system. The 2001 election of northern populist Thaksin Shinawatara began a period of social discord from which Thailand is still struggling to recover. In simplest terms this is a consensus society which has been unable to come to consensus. Thaksin or his proxies have won the last three consecutive popular elections. He was the first prime minister in decades to win an absolute majority and govern without the need for coalition partners. His support was primarily drawn from the northern region, including his native Chiang Mai, and from the populous northeast, Issan, the agricultural heartland of the Thai state. A telecom billionaire, and an authoritarian in style and action, he nonetheless delivered for the rural and urban working people who supported him, with a popular universal health coverage scheme, favorable terms for rice farmers, and a willingness to challenge old elites. Those elites included the upper classes – moneyed Bangkok, royalist supporters, and many of the more educated and democratically oriented middle class, who found Thaksin's populism and corruption abhorrent.

Thai society had wildly differing views of Khun Thaksin, from fervent love to equally fervent disdain. The vaunted Thai consensus began to fray in his first term in power. He was reelected, again with a large plurality, in 2005. Charged with a land grab corruption scheme, Thaksin was forced to flee the kingdom after a military coup in 2006 and has not yet been able to return. But instability worsened after his ouster. The country was soon wracked by protests, and eventually, outright violence between his Red Shirt supporters and Yellow Shirt opponents. The military intervened, with considerable loss of (largely Red Shirt) life, in 2010. In the subsequent popular election of 2011 Thaksin's younger sister, Yingluck Shinawatara, won a resounding victory, despite having no political experience. But the old elites, ominously including the military, could not tolerate a Thaksin proxy. Khun Yingluck was removed from power in the 2014 coup d'état led by General Prayuth Chan-Ocha, now the prime minister. And so in 2016 Thailand is again under military rule, the social split remains unresolved, and all signs indicate that given a fair election, Thaksin would likely do well again. That may mean a fair election is unlikely.

If Thailand has gone backwards to military rule, Burma, to the world's astonishment, began a political transformation in 2011 which is still unfolding. This was not the outcome of a popular uprising, but rather a 'top-down' move initiated by the generals after more than 50 years of junta rule. The unexpected opening culminated in 2015 general elections won handily, for the second time in Burmese history, by Daw Aung San Suu Kyi and her National League for Democracy. Denied the presidency (as she had been after her 1990 victory) by a military drafted constitution, she is nonetheless at last the acknowledged leader of her country. And Burma is in the thick of a rapid, unsteady, but undeniable transition from the shut tight authoritarian state of the past.

Such changes have eluded the people of Laos. She was, and remains, the world's only Marxist-Leninist Buddhist state – still governed by a small, secretive politburo, and still thought to be dominated by her much stronger neighbor, Vietnam. Laos is a regional holdout against change. HIV has never become epidemic in Laos, with the exception of spread among gay men in her cities. In September of 2016 Barack Obama became the first sitting U.S. president to visit Laos – part of his pivot to Asia policy. What major health issue did he address? One that still lingers, sadly, for the Lao – unexploded ordinance from the American bombing during the secret war.

Cambodia, then and now, is a single party state under strongman rule. Hun Sen, put in power by Vietnam when they invaded to end the Khmer Rouge reign of terror, still has a stranglehold on political life. But Cambodia is a much-vaunted success story in AIDS – and has received considerable international praise for the successes of the national program. This reality raises an old conundrum in public health: vertical programs, those focused on a single disease or problem, *can* work. But they don't necessarily improve health outcomes in other areas – or mark overall improvements in well-being. This is especially true when a vertical program, like the HIV response in Cambodia, has been largely externally funded. There is a long history of such programs demonstrating great results – until the donor money dries up. Nevertheless, Cambodia is on track, or so it's claimed, of being 'AIDS Free' by 2030.

Vietnam's recent history and her HIV experience have been unique in the region. The only country included in PEPFAR at the program's start, it was also the only country in the program with an HIV epidemic primarily among people who inject drugs. The country had been using detention, forced detox, and forced labor (borrowed, ideologically at least, from China's 'rehabilitation through labor' practices) to compel drug users to quit. This did little to address substance use, and nothing to address HIV, though it did lead to an extensive detention system of free (slave) labor which made many rich. With PEPFAR, the Global Fund, and the increased international scrutiny these programs brought, the ruling party were willing to shift the program toward needle and syringe exchange, methadone, and outpatient detox. Vietnam remains a single party socialist state, but one with an impressive ability to respond to threats, and to tolerate reforms which don't threaten the leadership.

Malaysia too, has seen some remarkable reforms in drug treatment, harm reduction, and other much needed policy reforms. But the political life of the country is currently ensnared in a battle over spectacular corruption charges against Prime Minister Najib Razak.

Someone deposited $681 million in the PM's personal account, and though the Saudi royal family has claimed responsibility, much remains unclear. Razak's party, the United Malay National Organization, UMNO, has been in power since independence in 1957 – and seems likely to stay there for some time. Political life for this sophisticated people remains stifled.

Yunnan's HIV epidemic continued unabated and unchecked through the 1990s and into the early 2000s. What had been an isolated outbreak among ethnic minority drugs users along the Burma border, extended relentlessly west – to neighboring Guangxi – and north, through minority communities along China's heroin trafficking routes all the way to Xinjiang, north and west of Tibet. The epidemic was finally addressed when a brilliant young leader, Dr Wu Zunyou, initiated both needle and syringe exchange programs and a large and far-reaching methadone program. More about that anon. China's HIV situation is perhaps the most changed of any in the region in 2016 – and now is firmly established among the Han in China's wealthiest and most developed region, the eastern seaboard. Yet as we'll see, it still has profound connections to Southeast Asia.

PART ONE

COUNTRIES

1 | COMING INTO THE REGION

1997

Highway 107 runs due north from Chiang Mai, Thailand's second largest city, and for 700 years the gateway to the fabled Golden Triangle, to Fang, a trading town just short of the northern border with Burma. Chiang Mai is circled by a ring road which peels off several highways, including 107. Driving along the stretch inside the ring road, lined with shopping malls and discount outlets, truck depots, and shiny new gas stations, it's easy to agree with the Thais that their modern kingdom can hardly be called 'developing' or 'Third World': the ring around the old city is as thoroughly developed as it is unattractive. Stuck with you in the ubiquitous traffic are a seemingly impossible number of late model cars – Mercedes Benz's, BMWs, Mitsubishi Land Rovers, Pajero jeeps. A decade of double-digit annual economic growth has generated real, if unevenly distributed, wealth. Once you take the turn north, the communities that support both the shopping arcades and the first-class traffic begin to appear. Suburban Chiang Mai was once mostly fruit orchards and paddy fields, scattered farming communities and country *wats* (temples). Much of it was forest. You can still see some fruit trees, even the occasional paddy, but what predominates are sprawling housing developments, condominium sub-divisions, and golf courses. Take away the transplanted palms and the odd Thai touch to a roof gable, and you could be heading north out of Fort Lauderdale or Atlanta. The old-style Thai houses that remain along the road, their dark teak frames beaten down by monsoons and the potent northern sun, look fragile and transitory scattered among the developments, like memories already half-forgotten.

As you leave Chiang Mai behind, heading north out of the valley of the Ping River, the balance between new and old, rich and poor, starts to shift. After about 60 kilometers the condos cease, cattle appear, and water buffaloes, fields of bean and garlic. Houses are more and more of wood, less prosperous, fewer. Soon after you come to Chiang Dao, Mountain of Stars, a single limestone crag that announces the coming climb. The mountains here are not high, the peaks are all under 5,000 feet, but they are densely packed and steep, the eastern-most tail of the Himalayas. The forest cover is secondary or tertiary, the teak stands are a memory, like the elephant herds that foraged here till the 1930s. The town of Chiang Dao, nestled in these crags, is easy to miss; the major employer is an army camp, and the service sector around it, which includes a half-dozen or so cheap brothels, some beer halls, a video parlor.

From here to Fang it's another 200 kilometers of mountains falling to hills, narrow valleys cut by the Ping, occasional villages. The traffic is long gone; people up here are on motorcycles, or packed to standing in the back of pick-ups. Many are not Thai. You find Hmong, Lisu, Lahu, and Akha tribespeople in these districts. The men dressed like Thai farmers, the women a rainbow of richly colored cloths, elaborate headdresses, the babies they carry bundles bright as birds.

Coming into Fang after the drive is something of a disappointment. The town, a smallish farming and trading post, simply starts, without any obvious relation to the hills behind it. Most of the buildings are concrete block shophouses built along either side of Highway 107. There's a bus station, a truck depot, a disproportionate number of banks. The Burmese border is still 25 kilometers further north. The place has little to offer the tourist or traveler – most pass right through it heading for Thaton, where the twisty Kok River comes out of Burma and runs east to Chiang Rai, on the base of the Golden Triangle. Boat trips on the Kok are popular, the scenery lovely; paddy fields and banana groves along the shore give way to rolling green foothills, and they to bluish mountains in the distance. The first time I went to Fang, shortly after moving to Thailand in 1992, I went with two nurses from the Thai Ministry of Public Health and a professor from Chiang Mai University. Fang was going to be one of our study sites for a research project on HIV, the virus that causes AIDS.[1] Though Fang is about as far from bustling Bangkok, the Thai capital, as you can go and still be in Thailand, the district had already reported astonishingly high rates of HIV infection among its farmers and traders. The 25-bed district hospital was fast becoming an AIDS care center; close to half the admissions were for HIV-related illnesses. Despite its seeming isolation, and the lazy rural air of Fang's dozen or so dusty streets, the community was going to be as hard hit as San Francisco or Kinshasa.

We were met in the hospital parking lot by the director, a smiling man in his late thirties named Dr Samadjarn, thankfully fluent in English. He and seven nurses were clinical staff of the hospital. We sat down to tea and pleasantries, introductions were made all around, and friends and colleagues asked after. The atmosphere, new to me then and ever after a delight, was warm, polite but engaging, calm yet energized, more like a reunion of old friends than a medical meeting. The Fang staff were eager to be part of our project. It was soon clear to us all that they could do what we were asking, that they wanted to know more, to do more. It was also clear that the staff from Chiang Mai and from Fang had already agreed to the collaboration – the visit was a formality, but an essential one; we had to know each other and we had to visit their district if we were going to work together. The hard parts – negotiations, budgets, staff assignments – had been worked out well in advance of our trip.

When the meeting was over, we toured the facilities. The in-patient ward was full; it would always be so when we returned. There were three patients getting intravenous drips of amphotericin B, an anti-fungal drug used in AIDS: two men and a woman, all farmers, and all with the same disease, *penicillosis* – a blood, multi-organ and skin infection caused by a fungus of extreme rarity outside this region, but common among people with AIDS in these hills. (It causes unmistakable black-centered lesions on the skin; untreated, it is uniformly fatal.) The hospital had a basic lab, two private counseling rooms, an STD (sexually transmitted disease) clinic, an x-ray machine. Everything was fairly simple but clean and functioning. The outpatient service had an open-air waiting room with several rows of long wooden benches under a fiberglass roof. We were a welcome distraction from the wait – a white face was clearly novel – much pointing and giggling went on, children hiding behind their mothers, bubbles of talk. They seemed to be poor, rural people, like their neighbors with AIDS on the ward, Thais and a mix of tribal minorities in their distinctive costumes. The nurses called them *Chao Kow*, people of the mountains.

In the afternoon we were taken on a tour of the district. Dr Samadjarn was not from Fang; he'd been assigned to the hospital by the government, but he'd come to know the area well. We drove out of town and into the low hills off to the west, toward Burma. Scattered villages, fields, orchards of mango and litchi, small herds of thin, long-eared Brahma cattle. The road followed a branch of the Kok higher into the hills. We turned off it quite suddenly and veered steeply down into a wide, shallow valley. A manicured valley of orange trees, row upon row of them, filling the floor right to its steep walls and rolling back up it almost out of sight. In the distance, beyond the groves, was a cement dam. Above it, a large reservoir had been built to hold water for the trees. 'The second largest citrus orchard in Southeast Asia', said Dr Samadjarn, with some pride. The orchard (and its dam and processing plant) was a foreign-funded development project making orange-juice concentrate for export. There were a good many workers among the rows, men and women in wide straw hats and huge floppy rubber boots, spraying insecticide out of metal drums strapped on their backs. It looked like hot work.

We stopped for sodas in the home of the owner, a large structure of gleaming golden teak, built in the old Thai style but clearly very new. Then Dr Samadjarn suggested we visit a nearby village. There was a family there he needed to visit, and whom he wanted us to meet. Their village, about five kilometers downriver from the orchard, was also new, but it wasn't built in any style – cheap tin-roofed shacks, several little palm-thatched shops selling cigarettes, soap, whiskey, a few low concrete houses, and, unusually for a Thai village, no *wat*. The place, we learned, was actually the result of the relocation of three older villages. These had been drowned out when the dam went up, and the villagers moved here.

We parked our van in some shade near the road and walked through the village on a dirt track, dry and hard in this season. There were few people moving. Most of the able-bodied were away, working in the orchard or farther afield. In the front yards of the houses, tending small gardens or sitting in shade, were some older people and young children. On the far end of the settlement, almost to the hills at its back, we stopped at a small house hidden behind some tangled vines. An elderly couple were sitting on plastic mats spread on the ground beside the house, a ramshackle structure which looked completely dark inside. The woman smiled warmly and *wai*-ed[2] Dr Samadjarn as we approached. They spoke for a few moments, the old lady puffing away on a thick, pungent cigar. The old man seemed lost in a dream, and never looked our way. I noticed a boy of about eight or nine, very thin and dark, carrying a baby in his arms. He was standing about 20 feet behind the old people, peering from beside a tree. When I smiled at him he moved carefully off towards the house, dropping the baby with the old lady on his way. They were all in rags; the boy in just a pair of stained, ashy shorts, the baby naked, the old lady in a faded sarong, the old man in a pair of green fatigue trousers black with grime, his gaunt chest laced with tattoos. A few minutes later a man of about 30 appeared, in a tee-shirt and gym shorts, stumbling out of the house into the sharp sunlight. He looked thin, though handsome, a larger version of his son. His eyes, when he stood closer, were yellow and watery. The man, the father of the two boys and the son of the old couple, greeted Dr Samadjarn with obvious pleasure and warmth. He shouted to the boy who ran off and came back with a teapot full of water and some glasses. We drank the water standing, while Dr Samadjarn and the young man spoke at length. One of the nurses picked up the baby, who flopped in her arms half-asleep. The baby looked pale against her skin, his proportions not right: head too large, limbs too thin, belly tense. Dr Samadjarn handed the man a white paper bag, and spoke to me in English, which he assured me none of them understood.

This man was one of my first AIDS patients. Clinically he is doing fairly well, but now he has some depression. His wife died three weeks ago. This is the first time I've seen him since the cremation. The baby is also positive, I wanted to make sure he brought him to see us in the next few days. The older boy is alright; he was born, I think, before the problem started. I'm not sure the old people really understand what will happen. They are very simple people. The grandfather has senility, too, what you call Alzheimer's in America. The older boy is the biggest problem; he is very intelligent and seems to understand what's going on. His father just told me he stopped talking some days ago.

The father followed us out to the van where the nurses gave him a big bag of oranges from the orchard. He *wai*-ed them deeply, then me, then Dr Samadjarn. He stood waiting by the roadside as we drove off, not moving, just holding the oranges above the dust.

On the long, hot drive back to Chiang Mai I feigned sleep. The site visit had gone well; Fang looked like a good place for our project. But I could not get the older boy out of my mind – his dark eyes, his silence. He had just lost his mother, and he was going to lose his father and his brother. The family was already poor, and going to get poorer fast.

I had been struck by several things on this, my first home visit to a Thai family dealing with AIDS: by the curiously warm yet formal relationship of the father and Dr Samadjarn; by the poverty of the family and their community, so striking after Chiang Mai; by the massive orange grove outside Fang; by the squalor of the new settlement (Dr Samadjarn told me after we'd left that the village, which had perhaps 1,800 inhabitants, had two competing brothels and a shooting gallery for heroin users); most of all by the face of AIDS in this place, so different from what I'd known in Baltimore and New York, where I'd worked (and lived) in another AIDS crisis. No matter how much one reads, it takes time and exposure to realize the implications of saying, 'In developing countries the majority of cases of HIV infection are due to heterosexual transmission'. The difference was in the face of a young father knowing he would not survive to provide for his children, in the eyes of an old lady about to have her world destroyed. Most of all in the mute pain of a boy whose prospects were declining as sharply as his father's resistance to disease.

I've been back to Fang many times since that first visit. Our project there did go very well, so well in fact that we didn't identify any incident[3] infections. By 1995 Fang Hospital had a truly impressive integrated AIDS care program, with a visiting nurse service, even a full-time social worker to deal with job loss and AIDS discrimination. But I've also come to know other sides of Fang, darker and more difficult realities without which it would be impossible to understand why the district's communities have been so hard hit.

In 1994 colleagues of mine began an HIV prevention project in the brothels of Chiang Mai, Chiang Dao, and Mae Rim, a Chiang Mai suburb. About half of the women they met working in these sex venues were from Burma. My colleagues, social scientists, began with some simple questions: Where are you from? How did you get here? The women's stories quickly began to be repeated: virtually all the women had come via just three routes. Fang was a central stop on the largest of these. It was a center for the trafficking of women and girls from Burma to the brothels of Thailand. The women had other stories to tell; Fang was where newly trafficked women were 'broken in' to the sex industry. It will probably never be known how many women (it's in the thousands) have been repeatedly raped and brutalized there before the transport south. Highway 107 carries them to the army camp at Chiang Dao, and further south, to Chiang Mai, Bangkok, and from there to Tokyo.

Many of the people working in the district's orchards are Burmese as well, ethnic refugees and migrant laborers from the civil war raging just over the green hills to the west. They work for a pittance and have no more rights than the women in the brothels. Like them, they are subject to constant harassment from the authorities, and pay out a fair proportion of their wages in bribes to avoid repatriation. Fear of the authorities keeps the migrant workers away from health care, from HIV information, from safety. Some of the other workers are Thai farmers who have lost their land to the dam project or others like it, and many have yet to be compensated. This is what happened to the family I met on that first visit. After they'd lost their land, the wife had gone to work in Bangkok in order to feed the family. Like many northern women with low education and no work experience beyond field and market, she'd drifted into the sex trade. (Her husband knew this, but when she came home with some savings, they had decided to have another child.) And Thaton, the river port for Fang district, is a smuggling center, partly controlled by remnants of the Chinese Nationalist Army, the Kuomintang, who run the trade through corruption of local authorities, intimidation, trafficking, and heroin revenues. I knew none of this when I first visited, and little about an obvious, burning question: Why here? Why now? Why should a remote farming town have so many families like the one I met on that first trip? The answer, at least in part, was that Fang, and many communities like it, was no backwater as far as HIV is concerned. In the battle against the virus, places like Fang were on the front line.

2 | THAILAND: THE DESCENDING BUDDHA

No condom, no service, no refund.

To the wide range of Buddha images found in Asia, the Thais have added only one unique figure. Sometimes called the 'Walking Buddha', the image is actually the Buddha descending back into the material world after instructing his first disciple, his late mother Queen Maya, in the seventh Buddhist heaven. The descending Buddha arose in Sukhothai, the first kingdom in the region that is distinctly theirs. The Thais had migrated out of Yunnan and into the flood plain of the Chao Phraya river only a few hundred years before. They came to a region long settled and controlled by the waning Khmer and Mon kingdoms. The late Khmer style had evolved into a kind of Hindu/Buddhist rococo, with elaborate decorative carvings encrusting virtually every inch of their corncob *prangs* (the towers that adorn Khmer monuments). Their Buddha was a solid, broad-chested man, with a knowing smile and a wrestler's thick face and neck. The Thais, once they overcame their Khmer overlords, created a radically simplified style. The change is as abrupt as that from the gilt and glitter of high renaissance Catholicism to the austerity of the early Protestants. The new Thai Buddha, having left the celestial realms of Khmer iconography, steps lightly back into the world of the flesh. Because they saw the enlightened one as having overcome all contradictions, all conflicts, he is an androgyne, with curvaceous hips, the suggestion of breasts under his monastic robe, a face that is both male and female, or neither, and of surpassing beauty. The Sukhothai form is all fluidity, in stone or bronze, all smooth curves with almost no decoration to mar the sinuous lines. The hands flow into flame-like points, the face is serenely present, the stomach, when it is shown, is completely human, with careful and oddly touching attention paid to the navel.

This image is the origin of Thai classical art. Once rich, the Thais quickly covered their images in gold and decorative filigree. But the

Sukhothai root is there, in the best of their design and art. It is an image that helps define the Thais' unique sensibility and culture. There is the love of beauty, the acceptance of the physical, a shared celebration of the sensuous and the spiritual, the practicality of an enlightened being who leaves the heavens for the fields of the material.

The speed and vigor with which the Thais overthrew the Khmers and established a new kingdom, a new style of art and architecture, was remarkable. This ability to consolidate, to adapt, and to make amazingly rapid social changes is with the Thais still. It is perhaps one of the reasons that they alone among all the states of Asia avoided European colonial rule, deftly avoided devastation by the Japanese, and saw almost no fighting in the long Indochinese wars of the 1950s, 1960s and 1970s.

Humor, pleasure, beauty, love of wealth and ease, the delights of the table and the bedroom, these too are essential elements of the Thai way. 'Thai', in their polytonal, difficult tongue, means free. Thailand, Prathet Thai, is therefore the land of the free. This is not only an assertion of nationalism; it refers to a very deep strand in Thai culture: individual autonomy. For men especially, the right to live one's private life as one chooses, and to take one's pleasure as one will, is a birthright to the Thais. This is almost unique in Asia, where the prevalent mode in many societies is the submission of the individual to the collective. This freedom, again mostly for men, extends to sexual life. In the past, polygamy was openly accepted. While it is now socially frowned upon, having a second, 'minor' wife is common for wealthier Thais. As long as the liaison is discreet, it is tolerated. For private freedoms do not at all imply public acceptance. The public presentation of breaks in the moral code, such as homosexual liaisons, minor wives, selling daughters, is a social disaster for Thais. It is referred to as 'losing face'. To force a Thai to lose face is to make a fast and enduring enemy. But as long as a man's pleasures and indulgences remain in private realms, and these open secrets are not publicly discussed, no face will be lost.

This personal freedom, of shame as opposed to guilt (to use anthropologic terms) as the controlling social force, makes for a researcher's dream. If you set up interviews the right way, and establish an informant's trust in confidentiality and your discretion, people will tell you their sexual histories, or recount their past bouts of gonorrhea or syphilis, without hesitation. You can find out what has happened, what their HIV exposure is likely to be, in minutes. This holds true for men in the armed forces as well. In the Thai army system, being HIV-positive, gay, or even transvestite, are not grounds for exclusion or censure. On public levels, however, things can function very differently. The Thais hold to their national myths with great fervor; they do not tolerate outsiders pointing out the flaws in their picture of Thailand, the wide discrepancies between national identity and gritty reality. Walk around Pattaya, Patpong or the other red light districts of Bangkok and you may be shocked at how explicitly sex is sold. The gay bars with go-go boy shows don't pretend that sex isn't sold there, and the straight joints are just as open. You can pay to watch people fuck on stage, see girls shoot hoops with ping-pong balls, thrill to a line-up of Thai farm boys jerking off. It's about as exploitative a scene as anyone could want, and all the staff are for hire. Yet Thailand was in a national upheaval when a British encyclopedic dictionary (Longman's) included 'widespread' prostitution in its entry for Bangkok. Selling sex is one thing, making it public overseas is quite another.

Saying the unsaid, I have often had that awful sense, familiar to all lecturers, of losing an audience. Discussing data on northern Thai sexual behavior, for example, and pointing out that the numbers show northern Thais to be much heavier users of brothels than men in any other part of the country, I watched the audience glaze over with disbelief. If the numbers are believed, they are immediately blamed on the poor, the uneducated, or the hill tribes (who are in fact too poor to use such services). Bring up the same topic over beers, in a casual conversation, and all the northerners at the table will agree, with sly chuckles and innuendos, that they are the greatest party animals in the land. And of course, northern girls are the most beautiful; who could resist them? Why should one resist?

There were reputable medical authorities suggesting as late as 1985 that Asians might be genetically 'resistant' to HIV. The Thai epidemic later proved this thinking hopelessly wrong. But it was striking, looking at the AIDS map in the 1980s, that Asia seemed to be spared. Thailand was the country that first exploded the myth of Asian invulnerability to AIDS. This makes Thailand the logical country in which to begin an exploration of the Southeast Asian AIDS situation. The Thai kingdom also has been by far the best studied, characterized, and understood HIV/AIDS crisis in the region, if not the world. And it is the country I know best, having lived and worked in Chiang Mai, northern Thailand, from 1992 to 1997. Thai researchers, public health officials, activists, and people with AIDS have all been ready to address their difficulties, their work, and their hopes, with candor. And, although much of what is said here may sound critical, this exploration is also an attempt to repay countless debts to friends and colleagues, as well as to Thailand itself, a country I have come to love, even as HIV has led, inevitably, to studying its darker sides.

To understand HIV you have to deal with sex, licit and illicit, commercial and forced, oral, vaginal, and anal. This means going beyond 'cultural' standards and ideals of sexual behavior to study actual sex practices, however socially circumscribed. You have to look at the bleak realities of heroin addiction, the conjunctions of drug use and sex, and the role of the sex industry. It becomes essential to find out what is not working within medical systems, to look for limitations, to understand inaction. This is not muckraking, but the science of public health research; investigating root causes of the mechanisms of disease-vulnerability and spread in communities. Some of these mechanisms are common to all societies, others not. Thailand is not necessarily paradigmatic for her neighbors; many primary factors that led to the Thai HIV explosion and her impressive response have turned out not to be applicable to Burma, or to Laos. But other factors and mechanisms are shared. And for better or worse, the openness of the Thais to publicity about the AIDS crisis has also meant that if AIDS has an Asian face, for most people that face is Thai.

Waves of spread[1]

By 1981, when the first cases of what we now know as AIDS appeared among gay men in New York and San Francisco, the virus had already spread widely in Africa, Western Europe, and the United States. Because of its long incubation period and non-specific early manifestations, there was little indication of how widely the virus had circulated or of how many people would eventually be affected. The virus itself was not identified until 1984, the diagnostic test made available only in 1985. Once the test was available, and it became possible to identify not just people with symptomatic AIDS, but healthy persons infected with HIV, the extent of the epidemic became clear. Perhaps half the gay men in New York were infected by the time we knew HIV was present. Some countries in Sub-Saharan Africa were experiencing a new plague approaching Biblical proportions, with perhaps one in ten persons expected to die. These were the first 'hot zones' where the virus had been spreading in populations for an unknown number of years before an AIDS case had ever been described. Prevention of initial spread was an impossibility. Pandora's box had long been open.

Sporadic cases of AIDS also appeared far from these zones of early spread. All over the world in the early to mid-1980s, often in countries with very few other cases, men were coming home from Paris, Amsterdam, New York. These were men who had been part of the extraordinary international and interracial mix of urban gay life in the 1970s and 1980s. They were going home to small towns in the U.S., back to places like Thailand, often ill and often alone. The first known case of AIDS in Thailand occurred among just such a man, diagnosed in Bangkok in 1984. The patient was a Thai gay man who had had a long-term Western lover. He had come back to Thailand after his partner's death. His physician, Dr Praphan Phanupak, had trained in the U.S., and was one of the few Thai doctors to have seen AIDS cases before. Fortunately, Dr Praphan knew what he was looking at when his case first appeared. His patient did not live long. As far as is known, his would remain an isolated case, a spill-over of the gay epidemic in the West, a dead end for the virus.

The second case was identified in 1985. This was a 20-year-old Thai man who had *not* lived abroad. He was employed in a gay bar in Bangkok; a male sex worker (in local terminology an 'off boy': the customers have to pay to take him off premises) who had had multiple male and female, Thai and European sex partners during the 12 months before his infection was identified. This young man was probably one of the earliest cases of HIV acquired in the country. His is the first documented case of what researchers in the field think of as the first wave of the Thai epidemic. Several studies of male sex workers shortly thereafter made it clear that HIV was indeed spreading among these men and boys and, presumably, their clients and other partners. The other partners were mostly their wives and girlfriends, the majority of these men being heterosexual outside the bars and clubs.

The commercial scene for male–male sex in Thailand, in contrast to the extensive heterosexual one, has been limited to a handful of 'gay' spots in the country: Bangkok, the beach resorts of Pattaya, Phuket, and Hat Yai, and Chiang Mai City in the far north. While the men in the trade were, and remain, at very high risk of HIV infection, their numbers have never been large compared to those of women selling sex. Chiang Mai in the 1990s had 12–20 gay bars with a total population of perhaps 100–200 male sex workers at any given time. Add together all the brothels, bars, restaurants, Karaoke lounges and massage parlors where straight sex is sold and it soon becomes clear that female sex workers outnumber men by at least 25 to 1, if not more. The social and sexual network to which male sex workers belong is limited to perhaps a few thousand people. The spread of HIV among these young men was a personal disaster for them, a cause for concern for the health care community, but not, at least then, a cause of concern for the larger society. In fact, there is little evidence that this network was involved in the explosion to come.

The Thai government, through its Ministry of Public Health, responded to the arrival of HIV by setting up a surveillance system. Sentinel groups like sex workers, soldiers, and injecting drug users were screened for HIV every six months, starting in 14 towns and cities in 1989. Several earlier surveys had also been done by hospital or university groups. The information from these data would later be critical for understanding what was about to occur. Injecting drug users in the West were hit early and hard by HIV, principally because they had such limited access to sterile equipment and so were forced to share. Thailand was once a major heroin producer, and while this was no longer the case by the late 1980s, the country had perhaps 50,000 injecting addicts in 1988. Surveys among injecting drug users (IDU) between 1985 and 1987 showed either zero, or very low (less than 1 percent), rates of HIV. Then, in 1988, a dramatic change was noted in Bangkok. The sentinel survey at the start of the year found about 1 percent of IDU to have HIV. By August of that year, 32 percent were positive, by October, close to 40 percent had the virus. Perhaps 5 percent of IDU per month were 'seroconverting', going from HIV negative to positive, an unprecedented rate of increase. This was the second wave of the Thai epidemic, and it dwarfed the first. What had happened?

HIV, like any microbe, has conditions for survival and for spread. It is an obligate intracellular parasite, meaning that it can only 'live' and reproduce within a living cell. (A living human or chimpanzee cell, to be precise – which we must be, since the virus is.) It requires the exchange of certain body fluids – blood, serum or plasma, semen, cervical secretions, milk – to spread between people. It is, fortunately, not infectious by any other route. It does not survive in water; it cannot, as influenza can, spread through the air. It is not known to spread through the exchange of urine, feces, saliva, tears, or sweat. When its conditions are met, it will spread, with varying and still not fully understood efficiency. But it is a parasite; it needs its host, a living person, to behave in such a way that another person can be infected. We have to do its work for it. A group of drug users sharing needles without sterilization between injections provides an ideal opportunity. Enough blood will be left in a used syringe to spread HIV if the syringe is used again soon; the virus cannot live long in dried blood. Such groups are not hard to find in a Bangkok slum, but it is prisoners who are most likely to share scarce needles, and to share them with addicts from all over the world incarcerated in the same jails. This is probably what happened, since the subtype of virus (in this case subtype B) found among Bangkok addicts at this time was essentially identical to the virus infecting drug users in cities such as London, New York, and Rome. Once this virus entered the blood stream of one user in these needle-sharing groups, the others were being infected with terrible speed. Because the drug using networks were connected across the city and, eventually, the country, chains of transmission carried the virus far and fast. In a matter of months it reached one-third of all injecting users in the country. But how many were there? How serious a problem would this be? Estimates varied, measures varied, but a general consensus emerged that there were probably 50,000 people who inject drugs (PWID) in Thailand at the time of the HIV take-off, 40,000 in Bangkok, and the rest in smaller cities and towns. In very rough terms, this would mean that about 15,000 people had acquired HIV in less than a year. A large and frightening number to be sure, but how much spread would there be from this group to others?

With most cases still found among gay Thais, male sex workers, and drug users, the Thai epidemic in early 1988 still looked somewhat like a Western one. After the first two waves of spread, AIDS was still largely a disease of young men living in cities, men who engaged in behaviors that the great majority of Thais did not engage in, and did not condone. This was not East Africa or Haiti, where the great majority of cases were among heterosexuals, both urban and rural, and where more and more new HIV infections were occurring among women and their infants. Asia still looked safe from this perspective, and 'Asian Family Values' were routinely cited as having 'protected' Asia from the fate of the Africans. This rhetoric fitted well with the region's startling economic boom, and again, 'Confucian' or 'Asian' values of thrift, hard work, clean living, and dedication to parents, family, and community, were routinely invoked to explain the economic miracle of the 1980s. The economic failures of Africa or South America were failures of values, or so it seemed, and the extensive spread of HIV was yet another example of what was wrong with their social systems. The Asian way was superior, even if freedom and democracy were not a part of the 'Asian Way'. This argument was accepted with remarkable ease in the West, even when it was made by a dictator like Suharto of Indonesia, or an autocrat like Singapore's Lee Kwan Yew.

This complacency was not to last. Women working in the sex industry had been irregularly tested for HIV in Thailand since 1985. Some sporadic infections were found, but they never amounted to more than 1 percent of women screened in any sample. Until 1989, that is. A year after the sudden explosion among drug users, a similar rise was noted among women in Chiang Mai. Again, the rate did not go from 1 percent to 2 percent in six months, which would have meant a doubling, but from 1 percent to 44 percent in six months, a figure which seemed almost inconceivably high, especially as sexual transmission was thought to be so much less efficient than spread from needle sharing. Other cities quickly confirmed the Chiang Mai finding, though none was to reach as high a level of infection. National rates reached 15 percent of women in the sex industry by 1991. This was the third wave. The social and sexual networks of which these women were a part was very different from that of gay bar workers or PWID. This group involved the women themselves, their clients, and their clients' other sexual partners. It would later become clear that this network included the majority of sexually active adults in Thailand; it *was* Thailand.

To understand what was happening, or had already happened, we have to turn our attention away from Bangkok and go north, to the old kingdom of Lanna, where HIV may have entered the general population first, and where it would hit the hardest.

The far north

Chiang Mai means 'the new city'. It was new in 1295, when the King of Chiang Rai ordered it to be built for his grandson. The city was laid out according to sacred geography, a perfect square in the valley of the twisting Ping river. The city walls had four gates, each opening to the four cardinal directions of the compass. In the sacred, but not the geometric center, a huge *chedi*, or stupa, was erected, filled with relics, Buddha images, and protective amulets. On a peak in the first rise of mountains above the town, a temple was built to further protect the new city. This is Doi Suthep, and its central *chedi* was plated with Ping river gold. The inhabitants were a mix of Lanna Thai, a people descended from the ethnic Thai minority of Yunnan; the indigenous Lawa; and the Mons, an ancient Buddhist people from southern Burma, who had been brought to the north of Thailand in an earlier effort to civilize the region. The inhabitants spoke a dialect of Thai which remains the common peoples' language, a dialect peppered with Sanskrit honorifics, Pali terms, and the equivalent of thees and thous, archaic terms in central Thai that are still used in the northern language.

Lanna Thais are seen by their countrymen as quite different. If you ask a central Thai about the north they will tell you that they are 'soft' people: polite, graceful, and soft-spoken. Northern women are supposed to be the most beautiful in the land. They are fair skinned, small-featured, round-eyed, delicate. These differences are not just the stuff of popular opinion. Population-level genetic testing (using a technology developed for organ donation) now allows us to compare populations and trace relationships between ethnic groups. The northern Thais, it turns out, are related closely to the Shans of Burma, the Lao, and the Dai minority of Yunnan. The central Thais appear to be related to Melanesians, and are not even close cousins of the Lanna Thais. These differences have a very real geopolitical past as well. Lanna was only annexed to the Thai state early in this century, when the last hereditary leader, a 14-year-old girl called Princess Dararasemee, was married to the central Thai king. Until the 1920s, the journey from Bangkok to Chiang Mai took several weeks and could be done only on elephants. Tigers made the route dangerous. The Siamese tiger is now thought to be extinct, or nearly so, in the wild.

If you come into Chiang Mai today you will see vestiges of the old capital. The temple on the mountain is still there, surrounded by dense green forest. But it is a city of concrete skyscrapers, convenience stores, condominiums, shopping malls, traffic, noise, and dust. The ramparts remain in some places, and all the city gates are still there, though motorcycles roar through them day and night. Americans can have distorted views of this part of the world. We imagine an exotic place, mysterious and more 'spiritual' than the material West. After a while, you realize the locals see the same distortions. They see the city they remember, a city of tree-lined avenues, girls with flowers in their hair, temple bells, and elaborate festivals of flowers, candles, and lights. Bangkokians love to come to the north and visit this 'traditional' culture. They have themselves photographed in native northern dress. Somehow they don't seem to notice that the natives are all in jeans and tank tops, that the traffic is approaching Bangkok levels of congestion, that the air is blue with lead from the cheap gasoline, and that DDT has killed off all the birds except pigeons and sparrows. Modern Chiang Mai is growing too fast to catch its breath.

One of the mysteries of HIV in Thailand is that the center of the epidemic among sex workers, and later their clients, was not Bangkok, a city infamous for its fast nightlife, but here, in the more rural and landlocked north. By 1991, within two years of the rapid escalation of infection in sex workers, HIV was about five times as common among young men in northern Thailand as in the rest of the country. The fourth wave. When you cut off the upper north, the region we know as the golden triangle, the rates doubled again. It is tempting to blame drug use. Opium, heroin, the Vietnam era, more mystery and sinister exotica cross the mind. But the great majority of Thai drug users are in Bangkok, not in the north. The drug of choice for northerners, for which they are well known by other Thais, is not heroin but the bitter-sweet rice spirit called *Mekong*. Unraveling this seeming paradox was one of our first tasks in understanding the spread of HIV in this old kingdom. This is the kind of challenge for which epidemiology was designed.

In the late 1990s, the provinces with the highest HIV burden in the country were rural Payao, Lamphun, Chiang Rai, and Chiang Mai, all contiguous and all in the far north of the country. The provinces lag in development, and are still largely agricultural and comparatively poor. In 1991, roughly 4 percent of young men drafted into the Thai Army from the upper north were HIV-infected, while among draftees in Bangkok, only 1 in 50 was HIV-positive. Indeed, the upper north, with less than a tenth of the national population, accounted for more than one third of HIV infections and almost half of Thailand's AIDS deaths by 1994. Working with Thai Army conscripts, a large population of 21-year-old men, has helped to unravel this geographic finding. Northern Thai men, we found, usually begin their sexual lives in brothels. Older brothers, or other relatives and friends, take boys of 14 and over to the cheap local brothels which are everywhere in the north. Brothel-going is a men's group activity; it is considered 'perverse' or 'dirty' to go alone. Lanna men usually end up at brothels after a night's drinking, on payday, or during festivals and holidays. We found a direct relationship between frequency of brothel visits and risk of being HIV-positive among the army conscripts. Men who did not go to brothels (a small minority, perhaps 15 percent) were much less likely to be positive. The factors associated with HIV among these men, in addition to brothel-going, were not using condoms, alcohol use, having had other sexually transmitted diseases, and having had sex with more than one other man. The heavy representation of northern women in the brothels, cafes, and massage parlors throughout the country turned out to be another key factor. While making up less than one-tenth of the Thai population, northern women make up more than one-third of the country's sex workers (although this is changing rapidly, as we shall see). What historical and cultural factors lay behind these behaviors? Why were northern women so over represented in the national sex trade? What traditions were operative in sexual networks, in behavior, in the practices of the people of Lanna and in the status and treatment of their women, that had led to what was clearly a marked vulnerability to HIV?

For the northern Thai man in earlier times, having multiple wives and other sex partners was one of the privileges of prosperity. Minor wives were socially acceptable, and wealthy men might have several. Slavery was a part of Lanna life for most of the kingdom's first six centuries, and slave 'wives' were common for those who could afford them. Any children a man had with his slave wives were his to sell. The modern trade in young women no doubt has some continuity with this tradition. The current emphasis on monogamous marriages has been seen by cultural historians as an adaptation to exposure to the West; earlier northern Thai traditions placed little emphasis on monogamy as a virtue for men.

The social tolerance of Thai culture has also played a role in the development of sexual habits and practices. While social codes of conduct may be adhered to in public, and loss of face a compelling social control, Lanna culture has always allowed for a considerable degree of autonomy in people's private lives. This relative sexual freedom, at least for men, appears to have survived till today. The use of commercial sex services, highly stigmatized in many Asian cultures, is an acknowledged outlet for northern Thai men, the great majority of whom have bought sex at some time in their lives. Like nearly all societies, however, this sexual freedom applies much less to women. Social codes of female behavior strongly censure pre-marital sex, extra-marital sex, and multiple partners.

How then have so many northern women ended up working in brothels? Poverty is a driving force, and parental debt, especially from gambling, drug use, and drinking, is another. But these social factors are common throughout rural Thailand, and do not explain the over-representation of northern women in the sex trade. The social scientist Marjorie Muecke has suggested that an underlying cause is the old northern tradition of daughters rather than sons supporting their parents. Northern girls, under pressure to support their families, and often lacking the education and skills necessary for better-paid jobs, end up as commercial sex workers to support their families. This, as Muecke points out, is something of an ethical paradox. As a dutiful daughter, a woman sending money home is fulfilling her proper role. The fact that she does this in a dangerous and degrading profession only heightens her sacrifice. Yet such a girl is clearly living outside the social norm of chastity until marriage. Here again, social tolerance plays an important role in accepting these women back into the community. The fact that so many women who leave the sex trade can go home and be accepted in their communities is striking. However, this has had a devastating impact on these communities, as well over 40 percent of returning sex workers bring HIV back home along with their wages.

Could it be argued that in this context prostitution supports the institution of marriage? If a society accepts that young men are going to have sex before marriage, and that women are not going to do this, someone has to supply sexual outlets. The high value placed on female virginity, and the equally high value placed on male sexual freedom, virtually ensure that a class of women will be used for sex. These would not be girls of one's own class, or one's daughters or sisters, but in older orders slaves and concubines, in modern ones sex workers. One of the most difficult truths for many Asian societies to accept is that prostitution is a core part of their sexual and social systems. If HIV had not come along, the Thais might never have had to face this. What HIV revealed in northern Thailand is that the prevailing sexual mores, considered so much more 'traditional' and 'conservative' than those of the modern West, were in fact almost ideal for the spread of HIV.

Because the professional class of women who supply sex is relatively small, and their number of partners huge, they rapidly become infected with HIV, as we saw in Chiang Mai. The result is a classic epidemiologic situation: a highly exposed and heavily infected core group interacts with a much larger population, the predictable wave after women in the sex industry. In Thailand 80,000–200,000 women, depending on your source, interacted with millions of Thai men. The fourth wave was among these heterosexual men, among farmers, soldiers, students, fathers, husbands, sons. Between 1989 and 1995 at least 600,000 such men became infected with HIV. Thailand had undergone the fastest spread of HIV ever documented.

The next wave was both slower and wider, and was also entirely predictable. Men brought HIV home to their girlfriends and wives. Newly married women, housewives, mothers, pregnant women, fetuses, and infants were exposed to HIV as the men in their lives had become exposed. The virus had moved out of the brothel and into the home. This tragedy may have been entirely predictable, but has still been difficult for many to accept, so strongly had HIV become associated with prostitution. But there is mounting evidence to show that the great majority of Thai women with HIV have had one sex partner in their lives – their husbands, and have only one risk for HIV – his behavior, which they may or may not be able to influence.

Responding: civil servants and civil society

Dr Chawalit Natpratan is a public health physician and *karatch-akan* (civil servant). As Director of Communicable Disease Control for Thailand Region 10, the responsibility for government responses to HIV in the upper north has been his. That the people of his region were hard hit was clear to Dr Chawalit; that responses were urgently needed was also clear; that he and his staff would be able to implement control measures, and to have some effect on dealing with the rapid and incessant spread of the virus was not. But it would be telling only half the tale not to describe what happened next, for part of the story of the Thai epidemic is of an extraordinary mobilization against AIDS, and of some hard-won successes.

There are fortunate conjunctions in life and work, times when the political climate is right for innovation, when men and women of vision find support in public life. For the people of Lanna, one such conjunction was the result of a national disaster – the events of May 1992. Thailand had been led by a notoriously corrupt government in 1991, that of Prime Minister Chatchai Choonavan. He was ousted by a powerful clique of Thai military leaders shortly after. This was a complex but relatively painless transfer of power from civilian to military rule, a process which was not new to Thailand. But then the coup leader, General Suchinda Krapayoon, announced that he was appointing himself prime minister. Popular sentiment was strongly against the general. Protests spread quickly. In Bangkok, always the center of action in Thai political life, students and workers were joined, for perhaps the first time in Thai history, by shopkeepers and small businessmen, members of the new middle class. The protestors demanded that General Suchinda step down and allow civilian rule. The military responded with force, opening fire on unarmed demonstrators, killing a still uncertain number. Eventually, the constitutional monarch stepped in. General Suchinda crawled into an official audience on his knees to be shown videotape footage of troops under his command killing students. He soon stepped down. A caretaker administration was appointed to guide the country back to electoral democracy. This administration was led by a widely respected Thai statesman, Khun Anand Panyarachun.

Khun Anand fulfilled his mandate admirably; elections were held less than a year later, the military chastened, the country at peace again. He was also the first Thai prime minister to respond to the HIV epidemic. He met civil servants and physicians and listened to their advice. He created and chaired a National AIDS Committee, and invited a dynamic social activist and family planning expert, Khun Meechai Viravaidya, to run it. Together they scuttled plans for mandatory testing and contact-tracing, and instead focused on the rights of people with HIV, and on prevention and control. Thailand has a large and impressive civil service, staffed by career professionals, not political appointees. Thai governments and regimes have changed hands a dizzying number of times since the end of absolute monarchy in the 1930s, but the civil servants stay on in the ministries, the universities, the public hospitals, and keep the country functioning. These were people who, like Dr Chawalit, knew what needed to be done about HIV, given the political will and money. With Khun Anand in power, both were forthcoming.

When the first in-depth risk-factor studies of HIV infection among Thai men were published in 1991 and 1992, they were unanimous in finding that unprotected sex in brothels was the driving force behind the Thai epidemic. Unsafe commercial sex was a clear public health target. But what to do about it? Under Anand, the Ministry of Health responded not by trying to close brothels, or to arrest sex workers, but with a national program to promote safer sex. The '100% Condom Campaign', as it was called, targeted commercial sex venues throughout the country. Condom use would be strongly encouraged, if not mandatory. To make such a step practical, the ministry distributed tens of millions of condoms to brothels, massage parlors, bars, and nightclubs. Through the existing national network of public sexually transmitted disease (STD) clinics, sex workers were educated in condom use. In Region 10, under Dr Chawalit, every time a sex worker appeared at one of the clinics she (or he) was given 100 free condoms, along with training in how to use them. Signs began appearing in even the smallest and cheapest sex venues: 'No condom, no refund, no service'.

But outreach was also required. Dr Chawalit sent public health nurses out to brothels to meet the women working there, the brothel owners and managers, educating them and enlisting them in the fight against AIDS. The nurses, also civil servants, were the foot soldiers on the front lines of HIV control. Mostly middle-class women, they did much of the difficult daily work of safer-sex promotion, STD treatment, counseling, and handing out condoms by the million. Night-shift teams were set up, which visited venues during working hours. One team in Chiang Mai focused on gay bars, making late-night visits to every gay bar that would have them, handing out condoms to the men and boys, showing gay safer-sex videos, answering questions. Because sex workers kept different hours from most other users of public health clinics, Dr Chawalit and his staff set up a night clinic for sex workers. This clinic provided not only preventive services, but also STD care, counseling, and a safe place to talk. The government STD clinics began to offer free and anonymous HIV testing and counseling as well. These were staffed by full time HIV/AIDS counselors, male and female, to offer gender specific counseling. I worked with these STD and counseling clinic staff for four years and I can testify that the successes of HIV prevention in Thailand are due largely to their daily efforts, working with one person at a time, to make sex safer.

When there were gaps, problems, or areas of uncertainty, the government collaborated in research projects to clarify key issues. The research effort in Thailand was almost unprecedented in its scope and depth. The Ministry of Health collaborated with the U.S. Center for Disease Control in Atlanta, the U.S. National Institutes of Health, the World Health Organization, UNICEF, the Thai and International Red Cross, the European Union, and universities including Johns Hopkins, Harvard, Berkeley, and the London School of Hygiene and Tropical Medicine. The Thai Army medical corps established an HIV research program with the premier U.S. Army research institute, Walter Reed. When I was leaving the U.S. to join this effort, a colleague at Johns Hopkins joked that if you spread your elbows too wide in Thailand you'd bump into another epidemiologist. These joint efforts strengthened the knowledge base for interventions, gave focus to public health measures, and, importantly, measured their effectiveness.

In November 1993 our group was working with the Thai Army, measuring the rate of new infections in the conscripts. Until then, the rates of new infection had been depressingly steady, each six-month testing interval showed the same unfortunate finding: each year roughly 1 in 30 young soldiers was becoming newly infected. Sexual behavior had started to change; this we knew from interview data. Condom use was increasing, fewer men were going to brothels at all, and more men were reporting sex only with wives or girlfriends. But HIV rates seemed unaffected. As we analyzed the latest blood results that November, something had changed: only one man had become infected in the previous six months, as opposed to the usual 12–15. Six months later, we found the same low rate. I was literally jumping for joy in our lab when I saw that the second round of blood samples confirmed our earlier finding. Soon after, other groups were reporting what we'd seen; by 1994, a short four to five years into the epidemic, rates of new infection were falling nationwide. This was true for virtually all groups studied except sex workers, whose behavior may not be under their control, and newly married and newly pregnant women, that large section of the population marrying into a high-risk pool of young men, and starting families with them.

Possibly one million Thais had already been infected, but the rates that had been so high in 1989–1992 were now sharply down. HIV had seeded the Thai population, and infections would (and do) continue to occur, but at levels which suggested endemic spread, and not three per hundred persons per year, which, if it had continued, could have threatened the economic and social well-being of the country. Thank God, or the Buddha, for latex, that milky sap of the rubber tree.

The successes of the practical Thai approach were remarkable. And certainly they owed something to the cultural setting, to the people of Thailand, as well as to leadership and good science. Promoting condoms was not an attempt to restrict the sexual freedom of Thai men. The army had tried this approach – punishing men for getting STDs, declaring brothel-going to be in contravention of the army code – and it was a complete failure: HIV rates were unchanged. Condom promotion in commercial venues required the tacit acceptance on the part of the government, and the people, that while prostitution was illegal, it was widely available. This was one of the most practical aspects of the campaign: by avoiding a moralistic or legalistic attack, it allowed ordinary people to continue their sexual activities, should they choose to do so, but with greater safety and with the government providing the condoms. There is also that other ineffable but very real tradition of adaptability that the Thai people have shown in response to so many challenges. They were willing to accept the need for condoms, and to change that most difficult of all culturally specific behaviors, sexual behavior, and on a population-wide level. No other country, save perhaps Cambodia, has had such success with condom promotion or voluntary sexual behavior change. The only other analogous success would be the rise in condom use and declines in HIV seen among gay male communities in the West; a much better educated and sophisticated group, on a whole, than rural Thais.

This is not to say that the AIDS epidemic was not growing rapidly in Thailand, for it was, and continued for several years of mounting loss before it peaked. But we have to keep in mind the difference between new HIV infections, incidence, and new cases of AIDS. It took, on average in an untreated person, 11 years from HIV infection until AIDS developed, according to American and European data. Estimates for Africa were about nine years from HIV to AIDS (the difference being largely attributed to the interaction of HIV and tuberculosis in African settings). Survival after an AIDS diagnosis, again absent treatment, was generally about two years in the West, less elsewhere. AIDS epidemics, when hospitals were full and large numbers of persons were ill and dying, didn't start for several years after HIV spread had begun. By the time cases of AIDS appeared in any numbers, an HIV epidemic could be many years old, and new infections with the virus already on the decline. This was the situation in Thailand by the time HIV treatment became available.

This apparent split, between infections and cases, was and is one of HIV's great mechanisms of evasion. It also points to the unfortunate interaction of this pathogen with human ways of thinking and coping. Leaders tend to respond to proximate problems. The press needs disasters, overflowing wards, before there is a story. The general public does not respond to high rates of positive serologic tests the way most of us do to a sick or dying relative, lover, or friend. It is a testament to the Thai public health community that they were able to mobilize resources and programs for *prevention*, rather than wait until care was the issue. There were to be darker sides to the Thai success, as perhaps there are to any success, but Thailand still looked very bright compared to its neighbors. There could hardly have been a more striking contrast to the Thais' impressive society-wide response to HIV than the tragedies which were unfolding in Burma and Cambodia.

2016

Thailand now: sustained success and ongoing failure   The decline in HIV infections in Thai (heterosexual) men and women that was seen in the late 1990s continued. To cite just one piece of evidence, the HIV vaccine trial conducted by the Thai Ministry of Health and the U.S. military HIV program, RV144, required over 16,300 at-risk young adults and had to add a full year of follow-up to find enough incident infections to actually test the vaccine. The rate of new infection in this large Thai population was between two to three per *one thousand* per year. A tenth of what it had been at the epidemic's height in the north. Other sexually transmitted infections also fell sharply, by a full order of magnitude over the same decade. Thai Government condom use reached 60 million free condoms distributed per year in 1996. With colleagues from the World Bank, we did an evaluation of Thailand's success in an effort to see what lessons could be extracted for other countries facing their wars in the blood. There were many. Commitment to pragmatic public health approaches over moralistic or legalistic ones. The use of HIV surveillance data to drive policy. The vital importance of political leadership. The empowerment of affected communities, especially of women.

But not all HIV infections in Thailand or anywhere else are due to heterosexual sex. In the second and third decades of HIV in the kingdom her pragmatic and humane responses would not be similarly extended to other communities at risk.

The first evidence of failure for the Thai response was the outbreak among drug users. This epidemic, actually the first major wave of spread in the country, continued unabated as infection rates fell in the general population. The HIV sentinel surveillance among injecting drug users remained unchanged – at about 40 percent HIV prevalence each year, as did the policies the data were meant to inform. Why?

The most fundamental problem was the refusal of the Thai authorities to implement needle and syringe exchanges. The Thai Drug Users Network, a strong advocacy group of recovering drug users and their allies, pushed hard for reform on this front, but to little avail. As in the U.S. and too many other countries, the belief (for which there is no evidence) on the part of decision makers that providing drug users with sterile injecting equipment condones substance use, or even encourages it, was just too strongly held to be moved by evidence.

A second problem was the methadone program. The Thai program had a strong ideological belief (again, with little evidence to back it up) that methadone should be used sparingly, only after repeated failures of detox, and only in short taper regimens, generally of 45 days duration, until the patient is drug free and methadone free. What clinical experts in this area will tell you (and I am not one) is that this is woefully insufficient for the majority of persons with opioid dependency. They need longer regimens, and a significant percentage will need methadone for years to manage their cravings, stabilize lives upended by addiction, and achieve lasting freedom from dependency. With the Thai short course the evidence showed that by about day 22 of the taper, fully half of the patients were supplementing their declining methadone doses with heroin – the methadone was just too low dose to manage their craving and stave off withdrawal. By the end of the taper, the whole purpose of the regimen was lost on the majority of patients. And the majority were returning to injecting use – primarily because it is so much more efficient to inject than snort or smoke. With returns to injecting come returns to risk for HIV acquisition and transmission. An added threat to life from this approach is that users generally develop tolerance to opiates. After detox, tolerance is quickly lost. Those who return to using are at very high risk – overdose deaths after detox were and are terribly common. These deaths did not succeed in changing methadone policy or practice.

This was the situation in the early 2000s, when Thailand experienced a new substance use epidemic – albeit one from an old source – Burma. A street form of methamphetamine, a synthetic stimulant derived from the ephedra plant, or from its chemical derivatives like ephedrine, began to appear on the streets of Thai towns and cities. It was very cheap, less than a dollar a dose, sold as capsules meant to be smoked. It was potent and popular, especially with young people, students. Dubbed *Ya Ma*, horse medicine, or *Ya Ba*, crazy medicine, the drug appeared not to replace heroin as much as to bring a whole new cohort into substance use. *Ya Ba* users were younger than heroin users, often much younger, urban but also rural, and prone not as much to addiction as to escalating use and the range of mental health issues associated with heavy amphetamine use – anxiety, paranoia, thought disorders which could escalate into psychosis, and sometimes unstable or violent behavior. It is difficult in retrospect to know how common these problems actually were. But what was unquestionable was that the 'epidemic' of *Ya Ba* became a media, political, and eventually a social obsession in Thailand. Spectacular acts of violence attributed to *Ya Ba* users were staples of the evening news. In the public health community there was real concern that *Ya Ba* use would lead to increases in HIV risk (a concern that while logical, turned out to be unwarranted – *Ya Ba* users, who were not also injecting heroin, had HIV infection rates about the same as other Thais).

And the source? The sharp increase in supply of the drug was eventually traced to the conflict zones of Burma. The Wa, a powerful and well-armed minority group with a large territory in eastern Burma, had diversified their drug economy into production and distribution of methamphetamines. The Wa territory was under the control of the United Wa Army, a Chinese-backed militia with over 20,000 men in arms. The Wa leadership was on working terms with the junta in Burma, and nominally at peace. But they were arming, and they needed cash. Having little else to export, their economy was largely based on the narcotics trade.

The year 2003 was a watershed year for drug policy in Thailand. This was the year of Prime Minister Thaksin's 'War on Drugs' policy. The policy was largely a response to the real or imagined dangers of the *Ya Ba* epidemic, not to heroin use. The program was nothing if not ambitious. Thaksin vowed to end the drug use epidemic and purge Thai society of its suppliers and distributors. Some 600 people were killed in the first three weeks of the war. The BBC reported it this way:

> But the disturbing similarity among the victims – all shot execution style, their bodies found clutching weapons and bags of narcotics, and the fact that there have been no investigations into the killings – has raised suspicions of a deliberate shoot-to-kill policy by the government.

The policy proved popular with the general public and gave Thaksin a platform to demonstrate his power and control over the body politic.[2] It continued for two years, despite condemnation from Amnesty International, Human Rights Watch, and others concerned about the brutality, the killings, and the impunity with which it was conducted. In 2005 Thaksin was reelected with an even larger mandate than his first election. Yet there was demonstrable evidence that the war on drugs had also had significant negative impacts on Thailand's HIV program. This was best documented by Human Rights Watch, in a powerful investigative report, 'Not Enough Graves', released in June 2004. The report demonstrated the rapid decline in drug users use of health services as they went underground to avoid arrest or death – including HIV/AIDS services.

When Thaksin launched his drug war, or perhaps his war on drug users, he also started a second brutal populist campaign. This was his 'Law and Order' policy, which was aimed at Thailand's nightlife, and most particularly its gay nightlife. As with many an authoritarian leader, Thaksin viewed the tolerance of gay life, of homosexuality, in the country as a sign of weakness. Gay bars, clubs, and saunas were raided, shut down, or threatened with closure. In profoundly culturally offensive losses of 'face' the police drove gay men out of saunas naked, paraded them in public, and sold the right to photograph them to the worst of the Thai press. Most dangerously, the campaign targeted venues distributing condoms for 'promoting' gay sex. Condoms quickly disappeared from the venues. While it is impossible from the available data to make direct attribution, the two years of this anti-gay campaign, 2003–2005, did coincide with a sharp rise in HIV infections among gay men in the kingdom. Whether or not this disastrous policy was causative, the removal of condoms from gay bars and clubs could not have come at a worse moment for Thailand.

Fast forward to 2016 and these contrasts have grown ever starker. Thailand is the first Asian country to be declared free of mother-to-child transmission of HIV infection – new pediatric infections are vanishingly rare, as are new infections in women of reproductive age (sex workers aside). The country has led the way in universal access to HIV drugs, and manufactures its own generic antiviral drugs at low cost and good quality. When we look at HIV infections in military conscripts – they are sharply down overall. But where there are infections, they are almost entirely found in the subset of soldiers who have sex with other men. And here lies the ongoing challenge for HIV in Thailand. Her young gay men are getting infected at rates as high or higher than ever before.

The best data we have on this explosive epidemic comes from the Bangkok Men's Cohort Study, which enrolled and followed some 960 HIV uninfected but at risk Thai gay men, aged 18–26, from 2006 to 2010 at the Silom Community Clinic in the heart of Bangkok's gay district. The clinic, rather incongruously housed in an old Christian hospital, was the brainchild of Frits van Griensven, a distinguished Dutch epidemiologist who has spent decades working on HIV in Thailand. It was Frits's vision that prospective cohort data would be essential to understanding what was driving the extravagant rates of new infection in Thai gay men. The study provided what was then state-of-the-art HIV prevention, including regular HIV testing and counseling (every six months), regular screening, and treatment for other sexually transmitted infections, like syphilis and gonorrhea, and free condoms and condom-compatible lube. PrEP was still investigational at the time, but post-exposure prophylaxis, where a man might get on an emergent short course of antiviral drugs after an exposure, somewhat analogous to 'morning after' contraception for women, was also provided. The result? HIV infection rates were over 4 percent per year and did not budge over the five years of the study. They were highest among the youngest men, those aged 18–21, an incredible 33 percent of whom acquired HIV over the five years. And this despite a truly outstanding gay-friendly prevention program in a country with universal access to treatment.

This is a Thai problem. But it is also a regional and a global one. As we'll see in the case of China, there is good reason to say that the Thai epidemic has had significant impact on expanding what is now the world's largest outbreak among gay men – that of the eastern seaboard of China.

In an important step, the Thai Ministry of Health has approved PrEP for prevention, and this may make the difference for gay men and others at risk. But they have yet to agree to pay for it through the public system, limiting its utility to those men who can pay. At 900 Baht a month, about U.S.$25, it's not terribly expensive for middle-class Thais, but out of reach for the young men working in Bangkok or Pattaya. For now, this wave of spread looks tragically likely to continue.

3 | BURMA: GOING TO MYANMAR, BEING IN BURMA

Burma and Thailand share a land border almost 2,100 kilometers long, from the mountains of Thailand's far north to Burma's deepest south on the narrow and steamy isthmus of Kra. The Burmese and the Thais share long, entangled histories, old grudges and rivalries, and memories of great victories, occupations, and defeats. They also share Theravada Buddhism, the Pali canonical language, and calendars and traditions rooted in the cultivation of rice. Yet it would be difficult to find two countries with more radically different modern histories. Thailand escaped European domination; Burma did not – she was colonized by the British and ruled as part of the Indian Raj. In the Second World War, Thailand sided for a time with Imperial Japan, officially declaring war on the Allies in return for a comparatively moderate Japanese presence. Burma was one of the fiercest and most horrific theaters of the Pacific war, immortalized by the British who fought there. After the war, Thailand moved steadily toward modernity. Burma soon plunged into a civil conflict from which it is struggling to emerge.

By the late 1990s Thailand had become an international travel and business hub, its economy growing at 7–8 percent per year in absolute terms, its ports and airports among the busiest in the world. Burma remained a closed, secretive state. One is an Asian economic miracle, one of the little dragons of the Pacific Rim; the other classed by the United Nations as a 'least developed nation', arguably one of the poorest places in the world.

Times have changed.

In 2016, it is Thailand that is under military rule. A new constitution drafted by the ruling junta and supported by a popular referendum (and a muzzled free press and sharply constrained opposition parties) is seen by most observers as markedly undemocratic. The junta leader, now prime minister, openly described Burma's military-designed constitution as a good model for his own. For those interested in containing electoral democracy, the former general has a point.

And Burma? Or Myanmar, as the new government now calls the country? Daw Aung San Suu Kyi is the elected leader of the first National League for Democracy (NLD) government, with multiple portfolios, including foreign minister. The ultimate prize, the presidency, was denied her by the constitution's clause that the leader could not have immediate family members who were not citizens of the country. (This had been designed to exclude Daw Suu Kyi based on her marriage to the late Michael Aris, but in 2015 was based on the British citizenship of their two sons.) The Myanmar media now refers to her as 'State Counselor'. Nevertheless, change is undeniably underway. The sanctions regime has been dismantled. The great majority of Burma's political prisoners have been freed. Full diplomatic relations with the U.S. and most other world powers have been established. And an investment boom, if not yet a development one, has been intense. In a few short years, the old capitol of Rangoon has gone from a city of golden pagodas, threadbare wooden houses, and huge old trees to yet another sprawling Asian generic of massive shopping malls, condo towers and plus-size mansions. It now has some of the most expensive real estate in Asia. And it is literally choking on the new traffic, as cars are added daily to the aging roads.

But much has not changed. The Burmese military, the *Tatmadaw*, remains a powerful force in Burma. Their business partners, the Cronies, continue to prosper at the expense of an impoverished majority. The military held for itself 25 percent of seats in the new parliament. Its leader can dissolve the elected government with the stroke of a pen. They control the Ministry of the Interior, hence police, and border security. In October 2015 Daw Suu Kyi initiated what she called the 21st Century Panglong process. This was in honor of the long cherished 1947 Panglong Agreement signed by her late father at the end of the Second World War, and arguably the last time the ethnic nationalities and the Burman's had come to a political agreement. One year into the new Panglong process the military continues its campaign against the Kachin minority in the far north, with shelling of civilian populations, and violence continues as well in Shan State. The brutal policies in place against the Rohingya population of far western Rakhine State continue too – casting a dark shadow over the optimism of Burma's political opening. The Rohingya, disenfranchised by former dictator Ne Win in the 1980s, have been described as the world's most persecuted minority. In 2016, that is saying something.

Coming to any kind of political resolution with the military, the democracy forces, and the ethnic groups has proved devilishly difficult. The *Tatmadaw* is dominated by one ethnic group, the Burmans. Burma, however, is one of the most ethnically diverse nations in the world, with more than a dozen major ethnic groups and over 100 different languages or dialects. The complex 50-year Burmese civil war is also an ethnic conflict. It was into this longstanding political and humanitarian crisis that HIV entered and found ample conditions for epidemic spread. As nearly every aspect of life in Burma revolves around these complex political dynamics, a look at the recent political past is essential to understanding the unique dynamic of AIDS in this transitioning land.

Dialogue, devastation, and reform

In the early post-war period, Burma was high on the list of newly independent ex-colonies thought to face bright futures. Educational levels were impressive. The country's universities and medical schools were the envy of Asia. The Burma Medical Association, the first and oldest in the region, was already almost 100 years old and sported a proud legacy of medical innovation and rigor. The British had built an extensive railway system and the country had several excellent ports. While much of this infrastructure was destroyed in the war, there were foundations to build upon. The situation in terms of natural resources was even more promising. Burma had some of the world's finest hardwoods and was famous for her indestructible golden teak. It was the world's largest reservoir of jade and a major producer of rubies, as well as other gems. The vast floodplain of the Irrawaddy, coupled with Burma's ferocious sun, produced an almost ideal climate for wet rice cultivation. But the greatest resource may have been the Burmese themselves, a cultivated and literate kaleidoscope of peoples who were the inheritors of nearly two millennia of civilization; a culture of witty and critical poets, learned sages, philosophers, artists, traders, and farmers. Burma seemed destined for prosperity.

But the British left other legacies in Burma as they departed; there were unresolved questions of nationality and autonomy for some of the larger ethnic groups. These were non-Burman peoples like the

Karens, Kachins, Shans, and Chins, who had been the bedrock of the British forces in their war against Japan. The British military had been a virtually autonomous force in Burma, quite distinct from the colonial civil administration, a tradition some historians have seen as pivotal in the gulf between civilian and military structures that would later develop. The one leader who had succeeded, at least initially, in dealing with these complex issues, was the young Aung San. His murder, on the eve of independence in 1947, marks the beginning of Burma's descent into darkness.

Burma did not turn her back on the world immediately. Throughout the 1950s, despite internal ethnic and political strife, the country was a leader in the Non-Aligned Movement, and produced the first (and only) UN Secretary-General to have come from Asia, U Thant. But in 1962 this period abruptly closed with the *coup d'état* of General Ne Win. Burma dropped from the world stage overnight. The military ruled uninterruptedly till 2011, with the establishment of a transitional government led by former general, then president, Thein Sein,.

Ne Win, a secretive, some have postulated paranoid, dictator, set the country on a new path. His 'Burmese Way to Socialism' was about as effective an economic policy as the '*Ju Che*' of another regional dictator, Kim Il Sung of North Korea. Despite the boastful rhetoric of Ne Win, Burma's health care system went the way of most other sectors in the society: it crumbled. Between the loss of talented people to emigration, incarceration, and execution, and the drying-up of funds for public health, what many argue had been the finest medical system in Asia froze in time and then slid backwards.

There were repeated (and often unreported) civilian and student uprisings against the Ne Win regime, all of which were met with brutal state repression. The uprising against Ne Win in 1988 was different, however, because of its scope and scale. This was a national uprising, joined by virtually every sector of society. It included students, as had all before it, but also Buddhist monks and nuns, civil servants, doctors, and nurses, and even the long-suppressed gay community. The movement, known to Burmese as the 8–8–88 uprising (8 August 1988 was the date the junta stepped in and started its slaughter), was led by Aung San's courageous and charismatic daughter, Aung San Suu Kyi. She preached and practiced non-violent opposition to the military dictatorship. The aims of this non-violent movement were simple: the Burmese had had enough of Ne Win's hopeless and brutal mismanagement. Democracy was the key demand, the right to have a say in their own future.

One of the longest-repressed peoples in Asia had stood up. But the army was waiting. It will probably never be known how many people lost their lives in the 1988–1989 crackdown; estimates range from 3,000 to 10,000. Aung San Suu Kyi was eventually placed under house arrest – the first period of which was to last until 1995. Many of her colleagues and supporters were killed, jailed, or driven into exile. But there was a difference this time: the world, for the first time in decades, was aware of what was happening in Burma. Ne Win was reported to have 'voluntarily retired' and the newly reconstituted junta, calling itself the State Law and Order Restoration Council (SLORC), was immediately under intense international pressure. This pressure, and the SLORC's apparent (and mistaken) belief that they would win, resulted in general elections in 1990.

These elections were the first chance most Burmese had ever had to vote, and to give their verdict on military rule. Most of the opposition leaders were jailed during the elections, and could hardly campaign. Aung San Suu Kyi had no access to the media or the people. But one by one, all the time in terrible fear of reprisals, the people voted with their hearts. Suu Kyi's party, the National League for Democracy (NLD), won an overwhelming majority. Burmese still talk about these elections as a kind of shared miracle. Everyone had thought they would be alone in voting for civilian rule. So intense was the fear of the secret police, Ne Win's vast net of informers, that husbands did not tell their wives, nor children their parents, who they were voting for. But they had done themselves proud. A Burmese friend once asked me what I thought about God. I gave some vague answer about truth or love, and he answered with great intensity, 'God is the right to vote!' That was the feeling.

But the junta refused to honor the election results. After the bloodshed of August 1988, the people took not to the streets, but to the jungles. The ethnic armies, joined by students and democracy advocates, stepped up their insurgencies. The civil war began again in earnest. Burma's agony was to continue. Aung San Suu Kyi, now a Nobel Peace Prize laureate (for her commitment to non-violent political change in Burma), was released from house arrest in summer 1995. There was hope that negotiations to resolve the crisis might finally begin. But again the dictators stalled. Suu Kyi began, quietly, to rebuild her non-violent movement and the NLD. In June 1996 she called the first party congress since her release. More than 300 delegates (including nearly all the 1990 election winners) were arrested on their way to Rangoon. Those closest to Suu Kyi were swiftly sentenced to 7–14 years in Insein Prison, Burma's most notorious. Many died, including Leo Nichols, an Anglo-Burmese businessman and Suu Kyi's family friend. He was sentenced to three years in Insein for having an unregistered fax machine. Elderly and suffering from hypertension and heart disease, he died after allegedly being interrogated for 72 consecutive hours without sleep and without medical attention. The generals were still not ready to talk.

The SLORC were to last until 1997, when an internal conflict led to the junta's dissolution and the creation of the next iteration of military rule, the State Peace and Development Council, the SPDC. The SPDC underwent yet another internecine struggle in October 2004, which culminated in the rise to leadership of hardline General Than Shwe. His rule (which some observers argue has not yet ended) would be marked by harshening repression; the extravagant enrichment of the general, his wife, and their many children; an infamous personal animus toward Daw Suu Kyi; and the creation of a kind of totalitarian fantasy made real – his secretly built new capital city of Naypidaw, 'the Abode of Kings', 300 miles north of Rangoon.

General Than Shwe would soon be challenged by two events that were to prove decisive for the future of the country, one natural, the other spiritual. The spiritual upheaval came first. In August 2007 protests broke out in several places in the country over sudden spikes in the price of fuel. Buddhist monks marching in solidarity with the protesters in the central town of Pakkoku were blocked from marching by members of the military. Violence ensued, including the use of tear gas against the monks. The leadership of Burma's monastics demanded an apology. Than Shwe refused. The movement that became known as the Saffron Revolution was underway.

At first monks and nuns gathered in the several hundreds, including at the revered Shwedagon Pagoda, where Daw Suu Kyi had ignited the '88 popular uprising with a historic speech before the enormous golden stupa. Their numbers quickly grew. By the middle of September, the people had joined their clergy. They formed human chains, linking arms to line the streets and protect the monks and nuns as they marched. Everything changed on the day the monks arrived at the gates of Suu Kyi's shuttered villa. Her people had not seen her in years. The gates opened, she came out to greet the marchers and said one word, three times, which had huge resonance in Burmese Buddhism, '*thandu*'. Well done.

This shifted the movement from a religious uprising to an avowedly political one against Than Shwe's rule. The next day the people of Burma joined the marches in enormous numbers, swelling the crowd into the hundreds of thousands. Would Than Shwe back down? Or would soldiers actually fire on the revered clergy? On the people yet again?

On September 27, the slaughter began. The carnage, the beatings of monks – the cold-blooded murder of a Japanese photographer, were captured by citizen journalists and swiftly seen worldwide. For my Burmese friends, everyone I spoke to, this was a kind of final rupture between the governed and their leaders. The violation was profoundly personal. It also cut to the heart of the Buddhist nationalist rhetoric the junta had been espousing. These were killers of the *Thamma*, the Buddha's teachings, and of the *Sangha*, his followers. The image that many would not forget was of the countless sandals, the shoes of the poor, littering the bloodied streets after the soldiers had done their work.

Brute force would keep Than Shwe and his cronies in power for four more years, but the damage was profound. We'll probably never know the fates of many of the monks and nuns who faced the guns in those awful days, and in the months that followed. Many of the leaders were arrested and (in further violation of Buddhist law) forcibly disrobed. Many fled the country. Several of the monks who'd led the Saffron Revolution were from Maggin Monastery, outside Rangoon. The abbot, the Ven. U Indaka was arrested and would be imprisoned until the 2011 opening. Maggin had been well known in Burma for its large and effective AIDS program, a monastic extension of the NLD's HIV program. As punishment for the uprising, the AIDS patients living at Maggin were thrown out on the streets. Neighbors were warned by soldiers not to take these people in – or they would suffer the same fate.

The next cataclysm was a natural one. Cyclone Nargis, a storm of truly enormous scale and force arose in the Bay of Bengal and headed toward Burma's low lying Irrawaddy Delta. Nargis made landfall during the night of May 2, 2008. She came with ferocious winds, torrential rain, and a towering storm surge which proved to be the greatest killer. The storm took over 140,000 lives, most in the first great surge of the sea. It would later become known that the only preparations the junta had made were to secure the planes of the air force and move them out of harm's way. The people of the delta had not been warned.

The aftermath of the great storm was profoundly telling. As devastated survivors sought help, and hundreds of thousands lacked food, potable water, shelter, even clothes, which had been ripped off survivors by the shearing force of Nargis's winds, Than Shwe closed the country to assistance. The cruelty and rigidity of this position shocked the world.

Like many others, I tried to get a visa to join the Nargis relief effort. I wish I had the response of the Myanmar mission in New York on paper. When I called the mission to ask why my visa application was denied, the polite Burmese man on the other end of line said 'Sorry Sir, your visa was denied because you are a humanitarian doctor.'

As a frustrated world pressed to provide assistance, reports emerged of the relief effort underway in Rangoon, which had also been hard hit by the storm. Burma's 400,000 man army was idle, engaged only in guarding government buildings and the general's mansions. But Buddhist monks were seen all around the city, clearing fallen trees, caring for the wounded, mostly with nothing more to work with than their bare hands.

It took the personal visit of UN Secretary-General Ban Ki-moon to break the stand-off. Once underway, the relief effort, which grew to be the largest in Burma's history, was truly game changing. Many generals attending ASEAN meetings around Nargis relief saw for the first time how far their neighbors had come in wealth and development – just how far Burma lagged behind. What motivated the junta to begin their political liberalization in 2011 may never be fully known. But certainly the Saffron Revolution and this great storm and its aftermath made continued military rule difficult to fathom, even for many in the junta itself.

Freedom from fear

The first HIV screening programs in Burma were initiated in 1985, under Ne Win. No cases were detected until 1988, when HIV cases were first found among injecting drug users in Rangoon. Thailand had also seen an early spread to drug users, in the same year, but Burma would prove to have a very different pattern of HIV. The difference had to do not with the route of spread, for it was caused by drug users sharing injection equipment in both cases, but with radically different patterns of that use. Another epidemic preceded the HIV epidemic in Burma, and this was one of heroin use.

Before 1988 there were pockets of heroin use in several of Burma's larger cities. The bulk of opiate use, however, was opium smoking, and this was a traditional rural practice among several of Burma's ethnic minority peoples. The mountainous regions of northern and eastern Burma have several ideal climates for opium growing. The opium poppy, *papaver somniferum*, grows best in just such stony, moderate-elevation mountain soils. For decades some of the ethnic groups resisting the Burmese military had grown opium as a cash crop to fund their struggles. This was analogous to the 'war-time' economy of the Afghan *Mujahedeen*, who also supported their struggle by growing opium in their mountains (to which the West turned a blind eye, since the Afghan struggle was against the Soviets). Other ethnic groups were in more complex situations. Years of warfare against the central government had left peoples like the Shans without coherent leadership. A chronic state of warlordism prevailed in the Shan states. These warlords were supported largely by opium revenues. Warlords like Khun Sa and Lo Hsing Han became famous either as 'narco terrorists' or 'nationalist leaders', depending on who was talking. There were purely criminal elements as well, groups for whom the war was an end in itself; the isolation and poverty of struggle served their need for secrecy in producing what had become by the 1980s the largest opium crop in the world. Poor and isolated Burma, off the geopolitical map, became the world's single largest supplier of heroin, producing as much as 40–60 percent of the global supply. This reality was not lost on the U.S., or the drug enforcement agencies of the West, but they were remarkably ineffective in dealing with Ne Win, the SLORC, or the ethnic groups to curb production. The limited evidence available suggests that before 1988 Burma was a major heroin exporter, not a consumer. This was soon to change.

The National AIDS Program of the Union of Myanmar did not attend the Eleventh International Conference on AIDS (held in

Vancouver, Canada, in July 1996) but they had submitted papers, in abstract form, which were published in the meeting proceedings. One bears some scrutiny. It is abstract Tu.C.2547.

Rapid assessment study of drug abuse in Myanmar: A Ministry of Health & UNDCP co-sponsored project

Ba Thaung*, Khin Maung Gyee, Bo Kywe**. *Yangon Drug Dependence Research and Treatment Unit, **National AIDS Program, Yangon

Background: Myanmar society prohibits drug use, but acknowledges it to be a problem. In 1988, heroin use dramatically increased. IDU has since become a major public health problem associated with high HIV prevalence.

Objectives: To assess the nature and extent of drug abuse in Myanmar; To create a database to support a Drug Demand Reduction Program.

Methods: Used multiple sources and UNDCP guidelines; involved 36 high and low risk townships. Conducted case studies on 2277 IDUs in treatment units (DDTUs) and 937 users in 33 prisons. Also taped interviews, small group discussions, informal conversations and observations involving 186 key informers, 672 users, and 32 small groups.

Results: Drug abuse prevalence varied from 1.7% to 25% of township populations studied. Of 1333 addicts registered in 1994, 77% were heroin addicts, 22% opium addicts. 84% of DDTU patients and 65% of drug offenders reported using heroin, followed by opium (18% and 22% respectively). Users in DDTUs ranged from 12 to 77 years; 88–99% were male. Analyses considered ethnicity, marital status, education, occupation, drug preference, reasons for initiating drug use, duration of use, freq. of use, mode of use, forms/ dosage and expenditure on drugs, familial trends, legal involvement, consequences of use, AIDS knowledge, and reasons for seeking treatment.

The abstract is the haiku of science writing. You have extremely limited space in which to summarize your concepts, methods, and findings. There is a world of information in abstract Tu.C.2547, if we unpack it carefully. The great pity is that we don't have the paper, and this is because the researchers (who clearly undertook a massive investigative project) who did the work were not allowed to attend the Vancouver meeting. The same thing happened at the Asia-Pacific meeting the year before, and at the Yokohama International AIDS conference the year before that: no representation from Myanmar, all talks canceled, their poster walls blank. I did meet one delegate from Myanmar in Vancouver, a hospital official who knew little about AIDS and cared less, but assured me that SLORC was really a very concerned and good government. (A typical party functionary being rewarded for his allegiance with a trip overseas.) Whoever did the work you've just read, however, was something else entirely – this is some of the most detailed information on drugs to come from the government. Listen to the haiku and you can hear the drumbeats of catastrophe.

Title first. UNDCP is the United Nations Drug Control Program, whose methods have been adapted here. This is the 'rapid assessment' component, an epidemiologic tool to get a handle on the amount of drug abuse in a city, state, or country. Myanmar, of course, is the SLORC name for Burma; to accept the name is to accept the legitimacy of the junta; if you call it Burma, the Burmese immediately know where you stand. So UNDCP is working with the SLORC. Fair enough; their mandate is drug control. But there is a standing UN resolution calling for the restoration of democracy in Burma and for the transfer of power to the elected government.

In the 'Background' section, we have the first acknowledgment on the part of the government that the 'dramatic increase' in heroin use occurred in 1988, the year they crushed the democracy movement and assumed state power. They also acknowledge that heroin use has become a major public health problem. The association referred to in the phrase 'with high HIV prevalence' is, however, an understatement. Another UN body, the World Health Organization, helped the National AIDS Program to measure HIV rates among Burma's addicts in 1994. The result showed the highest rates ever reported among addicts worldwide: 74 percent in Rangoon, 84 percent in Mandalay, and 91 percent in Myitkyina, capital of the remote Kachin State on the Chinese border. Note that Rangoon (Yangon in SLORCese) is on the southern coast of Burma, Myitkyina at the northernmost tip, and Mandalay roughly midway between the two. The virus is everywhere.

'Objectives. To assess the … extent of drug abuse.' Given the astonishingly high rates of HIV among addicts, their number is essential to estimating how many Burmese already have HIV, but the second objective is more interesting: to create a database for a Drug Demand Reduction Program. This sounds, to those familiar with the jargon, suspiciously like the U.S. programs, always promised and yet to be delivered, to work on the 'demand' side of the drug equation, the intense craving of users for their drugs, as opposed to the 'supply' side, the narcotics industry that is typically seen as the foreign enemy (Pablo Escobar, Manuel Noriega, Khun Sa, the Corsican Mob, and so on). But we hear no more about this program.

As to 'Methods', 36 high- and low-risk townships were studied. This indicates the scale; it was a large undertaking. We don't know how low and high risk were defined, but we do know something about townships in Burma in this period. The junta had been relocating tremendous numbers of people and communities. These relocations, usually forced, had been done to move people off land for development projects, to get the poor out of the cities and into satellite towns where they are more easily controlled, to clear villages and settlements away from sites of historical interest for the tourist trade. For example, the premier tourist attraction of upper Burma, the magnificent ruined capital of Pagan, has been cleared of its surrounding communities. The residents of old Pagan were resettled, out of sight of tourists, in a dry, inhospitable area about 20 km away. These new towns are something like the townships and Bantustans of the old South African regime. They are often places of stark poverty and despair. The depth of this despair will become clearer when we get to 'Results'.

Do 33 prisons sound like a lot? And 937 users in these prisons? And then we have 2,277 IDU (injecting drug users, so we are talking about needle-users here) in DDTU, which we have to assume means something like Drug Detoxification Treatment Units. It is not spelt out here, but we knew something about the alarming conditions in some of these treatment units from Burmese who've escaped to Thailand. First, there was no real treatment. Detox was cold turkey, without methadone or other medications to treat the symptoms of withdrawal. Second, these were not voluntary units, but were on a prison model. Many were nineteenth-century jail facilities. The central one in Rangoon had undergone its first major improvement after photos of addicts shackled to beds reached the world's press – it now had running water. Conditions outside the capital may in some cases have been even worse.

Now let us consider the 'Results'. 'Drug abuse prevalence varied from 1.7% to 25% of township populations studied.' This took considerable courage to admit. If, in any part of the country, 25 percent of a township population is using heroin, you have an unprecedented addiction problem. This is one in four people. This means every family, every household. If most of the addicts are men, as we find out a few sentences later, then this also means something like half the men in some townships are using heroin. And remember, the HIV rate in addicts in Myanmar was then among the highest in the world. Look at the age range in the treatment centers, 'from 12 to 77 years …'. Another act of courage. This is not a normal heroin and opium use population. Twelve-year-old heroin addicts are rare in any country; 77-year-old addicts are unheard of. This age range suggests populations and communities where heroin addiction was as common as drinking coffee or tea. And then we see that 88–99 percent of addicts were men. This is not unusual, but it does also show that 1–12 percent of addicts were women, and 12 percent is high in Asian countries, where heroin addiction and drug use in general among women is rare. (The National AIDS Program estimated that in 1995 perhaps 1–2 percent of all adult men in Burma were heroin users, and 0.5 percent of adult women. An earlier NAP estimate, deemed too politically sensitive by military censors, was that 4 percent of men and 2 percent of women were using heroin nationwide.) The brand name for heroin sold on the streets of Burma in 1988 was 'freedom from fear'. This was also the slogan of the democracy movement, and the title of Aung San Suu Kyi's book of essays on democracy and freedom. What did the junta make available instead of real freedom from real fear? A deluge of cheap and widely available heroin flooded Burma after SLORC took control in 1988, and they have confirmed this with the publication we've just examined. Was the SLORC directly involved in heroin availability? If not, they managed to control every aspect of life in the country, every sector of the economy, save the most profitable one.

A student veteran of the 1988 movement now living in exile had this to say about heroin and the junta:

> If you put up a poster about democracy at Rangoon University you get 15 years in jail. If you hold a meeting to discuss human rights you get 15 years in jail. But you can sell heroin in the college dormitory and nobody will bother you.

Out of control

Heroin addiction does not necessarily lead to HIV infection: needle sharing does. When the SLORC assumed state control and began their systematic repression of the 1988 movement, they closed the country as Ne Win had done in 1962. Foreign investors mostly stayed away (with the exceptions of China and some Thai military investors who bailed the SLORC out of its initial financial shortages). There was very little medical equipment available, and what there was largely went to the army. Furthermore, having injection equipment in Burma is illegal (as it is in parts of the U.S., the so-called 'paraphernalia laws'). The outcome of these events and shortages was the development of a uniquely Burmese heroin culture revolving around the tea stall. Every hamlet in the country has tea stalls, traditional places for people to gather, drink volumes of Burma's strong black tea, and discuss the events of the day. Because needles were so scarce in some parts of the country, the tea stalls became local injection stations. Addicts went as often as they needed through the day or week to get their heroin doses from professional 'injectors', working in the backs of the stalls, or somewhere nearby. These injectors often had only one or a handful of needles; these were being used until they were too dull to pierce the skin, and then sharpened with nail files for further use. Hence the extraordinarily high rates of HIV among these users. (Other diseases can also spread this way: a short list would include malaria, tetanus, and hepatitis B and C.)

In rural areas addicts also made their own crude injecting equipment, and these 'works' were frequently shared as well; homemade needles were sometimes made from ballpoint pens, or carved from bamboo splits.

The syringe and medical equipment shortage was not limited to illicit use of these items. The medical system in the SLORC and later SPDC periods was also grossly undersupplied, especially in the civilian sector and outside the big cities. The underground Federation of Trade Unions of Burma collected testimony from nurses working in the public hospitals in the 1990s, which paints a frightening picture of medical practices in the country. Surgical equipment was re-used until useless. Disposable gloves were rewashed until in shreds. Rubbing alcohol, a common disinfectant, was in such short supply in 1994 that nurses were diluting it ten to one with water; it would smell like disinfectant to patients, but it would not be of much use. The NAP admitted that only 65 percent of blood was screened before transfusion – and even this low rate applied only to Rangoon. For the insurgents, the situation was arguably worse. They were transfusing in emergency conditions on battlefields where screening was an impossible luxury.[1]

Since most addicts are men, it takes little imagination to see how quickly HIV could spread from the injecting community to women. Another UNDCP study found that over 80 percent of male addicts in Myitkyina were sexually active, and 98 percent had never used a condom. Indeed, of the 350,000–400,000 HIV infections estimated to have occurred by 1995, the NAP reported that 175,000 of these were among pregnant women attending antenatal clinics. Since the number of pregnant women in a population is much more easily estimated and ascertained than the number of heroin addicts, this huge number is probably fairly accurate. If the transmission rate from mother to infant is roughly the same in Burma as in her neighbors, and we have no reason to think it would be different, between 42,000 and 58,000 infants have been born with HIV in Burma since 1988.

Condoms were illegal until 1993. They were an unknown item to most Burmese, who have had only the IUD for contraception for decades. Condoms are legal now, but expensive. A packet of ten from Japan costs 1,200 Kyat. The average monthly salary of a government worker at this time was about 1,000 Kyat. You could also get black-market condoms made in Korea but sold in Russia (with instructions in Cyrillic). These were cheaper, at 750 Kyat for a dozen, but to buy them would still mean not eating for two to three weeks. In remoter areas condoms were something the educated had heard of, but rarely seen.

What about medical care for people with AIDS? The first report in the medical literature on clinical AIDS cases in Burma was published in 1993. These were patients seen at Yangon General Hospital between 1991 and 1992. Most were IDU and most were men. Nearly all presented not with the usual opportunistic infections seen in developed countries, but with tropical infectious diseases like salmonellosis and tuberculosis, a clinical pattern akin to underdeveloped regions of Africa. A recent article on clinical care for people with AIDS found that treatment was essentially non-existent, and patients succumbed quickly to infections. A Burmese doctor working in a government hospital in a provincial capital told me what she had to offer her patients when they were diagnosed with AIDS: Tylenol when she had it and extra rations of rice.

In short, a health and human disaster, which was extremely difficult to cope with in the midst of Burma's political nightmare.

Being there then: 1996

Myanmar and Burma. Two entities that can never be confused but which, unfortunately for the people who live there, co-exist in one time and place. Burma is a place in the heart where democracy lives, Aung San Suu Kyi assumes her elected seat as head of state, and reconciliation starts. Myanmar is an illusion of power akin to Mussolini's *Era Fascista*, an illusion armed to the teeth, Buddhist Fascism, a seemingly unimaginable concept. Will Burma rise out of the realm of aspiration and be a nation again? This is the question at the heart of Myanmar; one cannot survive the *political* existence of the other. As for the two states of mind, both do exist now. The tensions between them divide the society like a mountain of razor wire, a barbed and bloody tangle.

Rangoon in 1996 was a city of deep poverty. The destitution of its people was all the more shocking because the people themselves, in their faded *lungyis*, patched shirts, plastic flip-flops, were so gracious, so deeply civilized, the inheritors of such amazing culture. You couldn't help but yearn with them, for their aspirations; but also yearn to know them, to hear them speak frankly, to hear their laments, their losses and their ideas. The reality then was that any such discussion could land someone in jail. Saying 'Aung San Suu Kyi', let alone that seditious word 'democracy', could cost one of these brave and decorous people their lives or their family's lives.

To kill time (already close to dead; only the generals and their kin were going anywhere) while waiting for permission to visit hospitals and clinics, I was taken to the zoo. You could also call it the 'Yangon Animal Torture Center', or, to be more in line with SLORC, the 'Yangon National Animals' Re-Education Center No. 1'. It was all revealed in the eyes of one of four equally psychotic tigers pacing their few square feet of concrete. A Buddhist monk, a *sayadaw*, approached me as I watched a pack of deranged dholes (the small, red, Indian wild dog) pace in their dungeon.

'You are a visitor, Sir?'

'Yes. I am an American.'

'I am Buddhism, Sir. A son of Buddha.'

'Yes, I know. Are you from Shwedagon?'

'No, Sir. From a monastery here in Rangoon.' Rangoon, not Yangon, and said with a very faint smile. 'Excuse please, Sir. Are you contentment?'

'Well, Rangoon is a beautiful city, but your people are very poor.'

'Not beautiful! Not so, Sir! This is a war!' He said it again, forcefully, almost hysterically. 'This is war!'

'Yes, I think I understand. In my country many people know Aung San Suu Kyi, many people support her.'

Just then some people appeared to be walking toward us. Her name, and the people strolling within ear shot, sent the brave man off at a quick unmonklike trot. In a flash of maroon he was gone. The truth of Burma was an open secret in Myanmar. Aung San Suu Kyi's father and the founder of the modern state and of the army, was still on all the old banknotes. His face and her face. The central market is Aung San market, the park beside the old royal lake is Aung San lake. Everyone, *everyone*, knows who the rightful leader was and is. They had already rallied for her, voted for her, sat through six long years of imprisonment with her, and some had died for her.

After a day reviewing incomplete, but still disturbing, health statistics, I went to walk the streets of Yangon. At about ten at night I bought a *lungyi*, a man's sarong. The vendor took me to a side-alley tailor's shop to have it sewn closed. The alley was narrow, unlit, very crowded. About two doors down there was another small shophouse. A young Burman, handsome and wearing tennis shoes, so not poor, stepped out in front of this second store. At a signal I must have missed, a crowd gathered. They seemed to have come from nowhere, but in minutes there were 30–40 people gathered in the road, poor people, gaunt and ragged. There were several middle-aged men in rags, a wasted young woman with her infant, kids covered in scabs – hair tinged orange with kwashiorkor, protein deprivation. Three very old, bent Muslim men were called forward and hurried inside past the young Burman. The young mother was chosen, and several of the kids, roughly, with much shouting and argument from the crowd. Then it stopped. Others pleaded but were turned away. Those refused stood staring a long time before dispersing into the dark. What was going on? A work crew? A job offer?

I paid my 10 Kyat for the stitching (the official exchange is 6 Kyat to the dollar; on the black market it's 131 Kyat to the dollar, a difference worth noting) then passed the shop on my way back to the main street. Mystery solved: it was a restaurant, closing for the day and giving away leftover food. The young Burman had chosen well: the elderly, a nursing mother, and the skinniest children. But at least 25 people had gone to bed hungry. In my worst-case scenario for the SLORC showpiece city, I hadn't expected starvation. (This happened a few blocks from where the Thai Central chain is putting up a huge marble-facade hotel, close to the creamily restored Strand, where investors stay.)

In November 1995 there was a water problem in the city. No official warnings came out. I was having lunch with one of the infection control staff and was just about to drink a glass of water when he stopped me with the whispered word, 'cholera'. Welcome to Myanmar.

Condoms were for sale from the betel-nut vendors. Walking alone at night, I was offered them on every corner. The Japanese ones were about a week's wages per packet. The driver the ministry had loaned me made 1,000 Kyat a month, and if the car needed repairs, he had to pay for it. Most months, it was a losing proposition. Sex cost 5–20 Kyat a go. But men who partake could be charged under the British-era rape laws: ten years in jail and a ruined life. A virgin in the best hotels (for the Singaporeans, the generals, the odd Chinese smuggler) cost 1,000 U.S. dollars.

Money was completely nonsensical in Myanmar. The notes were in 15-, 45-, and 90-Kyat denominations, since nine was regarded as Ne Win's lucky number and the number 10 was deemed inauspicious by his personal court astrologers. Like the junta, money was also everywhere and nowhere. The generals were not economists. Perhaps this non-system was the only one open to them, given their desire for both money and total state control. They were trying to keep a totalitarian political system alive, to maintain party control, but to have an economy based on foreign exchange earnings, tourism, international joint ventures, and the sale of natural resources. The result was a limpingly expanding economy, a new class of truly wealthy Burmese with state connections, no political freedom, and wildly uneven development. Health care continued to languish, HIV to spread.

The junta's biggest gamble, tourist dollars, led to a campaign called 'Visit Myanmar, 1996', and frenzied building of hotels, the forced removal of the poor from villages near sites of interest, and massive slave-labor undertakings to 'improve' historic sites. This had the distinct feel of Mao's Great Leap Forward, steel for steel's sake, with no real plan of what to do with it. So Rangoon had 20 hotels going up at once, unreported outbreaks of cholera in the streets, and a small dilapidated airport that could never bring in enough flights to fill half the rooms. It was central planning worthy of Stalin, with the same immense folly and social upheavals, which only added to the breakdown of the social system, the real local (subsistence) economy, the remains of health care, and family lives in SLORC's heroin-ridden new townships.

In upper Burma I met a doctor working in a hospital. He was a lovely guy: bright, committed, and brave. He was starved of medical news and information on HIV, and longed to share his work. We talked in the tacky VIP room above a local bar – his choice – a place supposed to be 'okay', meaning secure. He told me that in 1994 his superiors became alarmed at how many AIDS cases and deaths he was reporting. He was told to stop being so 'thorough'. His own practice had become almost entirely AIDS care. He was one of only two physicians in his town treating people with HIV infection. Most of his patients had three things in common: they were young, users or recovering users, and they had worked in the jade and ruby mines in Shan or Kachin states. This doctor thought the mines had been crucial in the spread of HIV. He explained that in the rainy season the mines had about 5,000 people. When the ground dried out, the numbers swelled into the hundreds of thousands. People came from all over the country to work in the mines. It was dangerous and most didn't do very well, but a handful did, and that was the draw. Heroin dealers were everywhere, as were cheap brothels; women migrated seasonally to try to earn some money as well. SLORC ran the best concessions; the poorest people sifted through their waste water looking for shards. When the rains came again, the miners went home, taking HIV to every nook and cranny.

This doctor thought the SLORC were not directly involved in the sex or heroin trades in the mines, but that there were corrupt people in the junta who are involved, and that their activities were tolerated because of kickbacks. The generals simply did not care very much about ordinary people.

Being there now: 2016

It is probably safe now to speak about what transpired on later trips to Burma. In 2000 Daw Suu Kyi was again out of house arrest. In that period, I made several trips to Burma, meeting with her each time. The first time we were able to have an extended conversation was at the home of the deputy leader of the NLD, Uncle U Tin Oo. She was nowhere near a free woman. We had to walk to Uncle's house, early in the morning, to be passing by around the time the security detail had their shift change, and we could duck safely into Uncle's house. To intimidate and harass the elderly U Tin Oo and his wife, the generals had cut their power lines, so their home was dark and stiflingly hot. There were two of us, and we had to hide in a below-stairs storage area through the long day until Daw Suu Kyi could drive over from her house to his. At about two in the afternoon, I heard her bright bell-like voice call out 'Hello Uncle, Hello Aunty!' And there she was, in Burmese dress, carrying a parasol against the sun, and barefoot as she crossed the threshold.

After some water, tea, and catch-up conversation, Daw Suu Kyi and I were led out to a side porch of the house where we could speak with some privacy – where there might be a bit of a breeze. I was to brief her on the HIV epidemic underway in her country, and what public health policies the NLD might undertake to combat it. As we sat down, I saw with a start that there was a soldier on the roof of the house next door. He was in a crouched position, with a rifle aimed at Daw Suu Kyi and seemingly at the ready. I gestured to her to look over, which she did with deliberate calm. 'Yes, they do that to intimidate. I hope it doesn't bother you. I think we're actually quite safe. Shall we dive in?'

In 1996, there had been a widespread student protest against military strictures in education. This one, as in the past, had been brutally put down. Once the generals were again firmly in control, they issued an edict. All university students would have to swear allegiance to perpetual military rule or face immediate and permanent expulsion from higher education in the country. Most caved, given that private educational options were few, and foreign education an option only for the tiny elite, the generals' children and those of the Cronies. But the young members of Daw Suu Kyi's party, the NLD Youth, resigned from the universities en masse. This was an enormous sacrifice for young people and their families in a culture that had always venerated higher education. Suu Kyi was deeply affected. Out of her concern came the idea of providing higher educational opportunities to the NLD youth with a radically different model. The idea was something of an open university, where scholars and teachers from a range of disciplines would come to Burma and teach several day intensives. The British political scholar Timothy Garton Ash, author of the terrific *Balkan Ghosts*, came to teach on transitions to democracy. A group of feminist scholars did an intensive on gender equality. And on that afternoon on Uncle's porch, Daw Suu asked me to put an intensive course together on HIV for the youth wing of her party.

Reader, I did not hesitate.

A painful but difficult reality of HIV at the time was the large number of women and girls from Burma working in the regional sex industry. By 2000, more than half the women working in Chiang Mai were from the Shan hills of Burma. HIV awareness was low, and infection rates high. EMPOWER, an NGO focused on sex workers rights and health, had a Chiang Mai office at the time and was almost the only agency working with these highly vulnerable women. Jackie Pollock, an English friend who'd been long resident in Thailand, ran the program. She had deep understanding of the issues facing the sex workers and a hugely compassionate heart for their suffering. I felt the NLD youth had to know about what the women from their country were facing – particularly the ethnic minorities then at open war with the *Tatmadaw*. So I asked Jackie if she would teach with me.

We traveled separately. Jackie from Thailand, myself from Baltimore, agreeing to meet only on the first day of the training. Since we'd be doing the training at the NLD headquarters, then under intense surveillance from the junta, we knew once we started we'd be followed, our conversations tracked, and everyone we spoke to, even casually, would be interrogated later about what we'd said and asked about. Since any educational materials might be seized, we had to do the training from the heart, without slides, handouts, or notes.

The morning of the first day was scorching. I wore my lightest suit with a short sleeved shirt and no tie but was dripping before I even got to the headquarters. It was an easy building to miss, low, with a sagging roof, looking more like an old car garage than a party headquarters. (The NLD had been denied all requests to make improvements by the local authorities.)

Looking for a suitable gift for Daw Suu, I'd come upon a flower stall near the Shwedagon Pagoda, where I'd gone for a morning meditation. Wrapped in lotus leaves and tied in bundles with vines were sprays of tiny light pink roses. Burma has gorgeous roses – mostly from the cool dry Shan plateau. I bought all they had.

Jackie and I waited for Daw Suu in the bustling second-floor offices of the NLD. Uncle U Tin Oo was there and very much in charge of about 20 NLD Youth members, all busy with party work. There was a rustle, a sudden buzz from the growing crowd we could hear on the ground floor, and then there she was, elegantly dressed as ever, and wonderfully welcoming and warm to us both.

'I hope you understand that since I'm currently barred from public speaking, I won't be able to address the audience directly today.' Yes, we did. And then with a wry smile she added 'But nothing has been said about serving as an interpreter. So I hope you don't mind my serving as your interpreter for the course?' Oh, not at all. 'Then, if you'll allow me, I'd like to say two things to the people here today at the start. Chris if you'd say them, I'll translate. First, I'd like to stress that it doesn't matter at all how anyone has become infected – all are deserving of our concern and our care. And then I'd like to ask that all are treated with *Metta*, with loving-kindness because all deserve our compassion. Would that be alright?'

I asked if she thought the regime had informers in the audience – if there was anything we should be careful about saying. 'Of course there are large numbers of informers at every event we do. I've been told about a third of any audience will likely be reporting back. So please just do your best and give everyone as much information as you can. The soldiers need good HIV education as much as anyone else in this country.'

And with that we followed Daw Suu down a narrow wooden staircase and into an absolutely packed room with perhaps 300 people. The dense crowd parted and went silent as Daw Suu walked to the front of the room. There was an intense sense of occasion that was hard to explain but palpable. There is an alchemy between a beloved leader and her or his people that is much more moving than meeting the woman or the man alone, being in the expectant crowd. I have only experienced this a handful of times – with His Holiness the Dalai Lama among a crowd of Tibetan refugees. When Nelson Mandela stepped on the stage at the International AIDS Conference in South Africa in 2000 – and the place suddenly burst into gorgeous African song. That was the vibe that hot morning.

As always, you learn a great deal from teaching. We met activists from the townships working on AIDS with virtually no resources. We heard stories of families being asked to pay for every lab test, every medication, even for bandages, at public hospitals which were supposed to be free. And we heard from many about the intense stigma, the shame, associated with HIV in Burmese culture. As people spoke about innocent and deserving sufferers like babies born with HIV – and about less deserving ones, like women who had sex out of marriage or homosexuals, Jackie understood why Daw Suu had wanted to share the messages she had. She'd doubtless heard this kind of talk before, had understood that her people needed to hear about practicing *Metta* – acting with compassion.

After the training, Jackie and I parted. She was due to leave that day, and I'd stay on another. We planned to meet up again in Thailand, but after she'd left I realized we had no way to contact each other if she'd been detained. This was a real concern, but in the event, she'd been fine.

Daw Suu had requested I meet her on my last day in country. I was to go to the airport after our meeting and then leave the country. She had a number of messages she'd asked me to deliver. This required the messages and the recipients be memorized, since it wouldn't be safe for her or for me to carry any written or digital records. After a private meeting with her, everything I had would likely be searched and seized. I went to the NLD headquarters and waited.

Daw Suu came into the office with a radiant smile of welcome. She had twined a spray of the pink roses I'd brought into her hair and was dressed, head to toe, in pink silk of just the same lovely shade. She has been a beauty all of her life, but that afternoon she was simply breathtaking.

My bags were at the small hotel where I'd been staying, so I took a taxi there. I arrived to find the place swirling with military intelligence, the MI. There was no pretense of being undercover, these were thugs with walkie-talkies and they had the poor desk manager pinned behind his counter and shaking with fear. Every other guest save myself had been expelled, my room searched, and my things strewn around. What to do? I'd been given the number of the U.S. chargé d'affaires (without full diplomatic relations, we had no Ambassador to Myanmar at the time) and been asked to call her when I arrived in country. I hadn't, as I'd been told by others that the U.S. phone lines were tapped, and checking in might have given the MI the chance to stop the workshop – or block us from getting to the NLD offices at all. But there was clearly no point in hesitating now. The U.S. mission sent over a car and a driver, and a helpful Burmese-American staffer who negotiated my getting out of the place. Still followed by several cars full of MI, we made it to the airport.

As expected, everything I had was rudely searched. I was soon approached by two officials in military green and gold, a man and a woman, both rigidly unsmiling.

'What have you been doing in our country?'

Taking Daw Suu's lead, I thought honesty made sense, since they likely knew perfectly well what we'd done.

'I've been doing a training on HIV and AIDS. Have you heard of it? It's a serious problem in your country, Myanmar.'

'Where? Who was this training for?'

'We offered it at the office of the National League for Democracy', I said the last words deliberately loudly, so anyone who might have overheard would know why I was detained, if I was. 'It was open to the public. It's so important that people learn about AIDS, don't you think?'

I did make my Thai Airways flight back to Bangkok. But for the crime of doing a workshop on HIV for the NLD, I was blacklisted from Burma for the next 11 years.

The next months saw Daw Suu Kyi once again begin to travel the country and rally her people to the cause of democracy. The crowds were extraordinary wherever she and her NLD team went. The people of Burma had not forgotten. But she was soon to face the most severe threat to her life of her political career. The regime was clearly feeling threatened by the charismatic (and democratically elected) leader the people so transparently preferred to their rule. On the night of May 30, 2003, outside a small village in the Depayin Township of upper Burma's Sagaing Division, they struck. Typical of Than Shwe, the attackers were out-of-uniform irregular forces. Armed with clubs, axes, farm implements, and some light weapons, they attacked a large convoy of NLD leaders, supporters, and the car carrying Daw Suu Kyi and Uncle U Tin Oo. The mayhem and murders which followed came to be known as the Depayin Massacre. At least 80 were killed outright, many more disappeared, some never to be accounted for. U Tin Oo dove on top of Daw Suu to protect her from the attackers, sustaining a serious head injury. Their car did manage to escape. The attempt on her life had failed. But both leaders were swiftly imprisoned, and this time Daw Suu was not put under house arrest, but held at Insein Prison. Uncle was held in a remote prison farther north, a cause for real concern for the elder statesman's life.

Daw Suu was not to be seen again until that day the monks arrived at her gates to ignite the Saffron Revolution.

While the 'international community' may be critical of Daw Suu Kyi's recent efforts at national reconciliation, we should be mindful of a stark truth. This is a woman who has had to negotiate a transition on behalf of her people with the same men who unleashed a mob of thugs in the night to try to kill her.

Many are skeptical of Burma's opening. Daw Suu Kyi has been criticized for her handling of the Rohingya crisis, for too close relations with China, for her seeming inability to rein in the military and its abuses in Kachin and Shan states. While she has been outspoken on HIV issues, real reform of the health system (one portfolio the NLD does control) has not started, and is urgently needed.

But some changes are palpably real. On a trip to the country in 2014, I was able to visit with Sayadaw U Indaka at his new monastery under construction outside Yangon. U Indaka had been the abbot of Maggin Monastery, and had run an NLD affiliated care program for impoverished patients with AIDS – until many of his younger monks emerged as leaders of the Saffron Revolution. He was arrested in the subsequent crackdown, imprisoned at Insein, and held until the release of political prisoners in 2011. During the years of his imprisonment I wrote and spoke frequently about this brave leader. I wrote his name on my office whiteboard, directly opposite my desk, so I could see it every day and not forget.

The Sayadaw turned out to be a thin and quiet man, about my age. A preternaturally calm presence. I asked him about the future. What did he think Burma needed to make real progress on democracy. I was surprised by his answer. Just one word, delivered with an understated smile: *Honesty*.

I ended this chapter in the 1998 edition with the short section below. My faith still holds.

> I believe in the Burmese people I've come to know, and that they will win, eventually. Buddhism teaches that all wheels turn, all karma ripens, all regimes and social orders, good and bad, eventually go.

4 | CAMBODIA: AIDS AND THE TORN SOCIETY

Cambodia is one of the handful of countries to have gone from a generalized epidemic of HIV – having more than 2 percent of reproductive age adults infected – to a concentrated one, where the virus is predominately found in key populations, like sex workers, gay men, and drug users.[1] The HIV epidemic in Cambodia peaked in the late 1990s, at over one in 40 reproductive age adults living with the virus. Spread at the time was rapid and the health system terribly weak after decades of conflict. Yet HIV was estimated to have fallen to 0.6 percent of adults in 2013, about the same rate currently seen in the U.S. and Brazil. Deaths from AIDS had declined dramatically too – to a third of what they'd been in 2001, as access to HIV treatment expanded across the country.

Cambodia had essentially no HIV treatment through the 1990s. Three years later, in 2001, fewer than 100 people (71 to be precise) were on antiviral therapy in the entire country. That number had grown to 46,000 in 2011, well over half of all Cambodians then living with the virus, and the proportion on treatment has continued to rise. Prevention of mother-to-child transmission has also been an outstanding programmatic success, having gone from about 5 percent of pregnant women being screened for HIV in the early 2000s, to close to 90 percent by 2011. These rather remarkable outcomes were presented in a plenary talk at the 2014 International AIDS Conference in Melbourne, Australia, by Mean Chhi Vun, head of Cambodia's National AIDS and STD program. He also laid out an ambitious program going forward to 2020, including the goal of eliminating mother-to-child transmission of HIV altogether. His evidence for achieving that goal was compelling. So was his sober analysis of the threats ahead for the next phases of Cambodia's effort.

Scaling up HIV services on this scale, even for a population as relatively small as Cambodia's (currently estimated at about 15 million souls), costs money. And the great bulk of the funding which made these achievements possible was from external donors, primarily the U.S. PEPFAR program and the Global Fund, which together accounted for some 87 percent of all HIV funding in the country by 2012. This generosity led to a striking imbalance in the health budget – while just 3 percent of the government's own health dollars were going to the HIV effort, 38 percent of all health dollars spent in the kingdom were spent on HIV that year – a serious donor bump. Given the devastating scenarios continued inaction and lack of funding might have yielded for the Khmer epidemic, it is hard to argue with Cambodia's successes or with the benefits of those investments. As often happens in public policy, you get what you pay for.

Success has proven more difficult to achieve in HIV prevention and care for Cambodia's still at risk populations. In 2016 these are primarily women selling sex, men who have sex with men, transgender women, and the small population of people who inject drugs. In 'Cambodia: AIDS and the Torn Society', in the first edition of this book, I focused significantly on the sex trade and the people engaged in it, since that was where Cambodia's epidemic was spreading in 1998. There has since been a great deal of government, donor, NGO, and human rights focus on Cambodian sex workers and the industry in which they toil, and on human trafficking, the large and growing entertainment sector, and on the impact of the 2008 'Law on Suppression of Human Trafficking and Sexual Exploitation'. Yet there may be more women engaged in variously described forms of sex work in the country than ever before. This complex situation is more deeply explored in Chapter 10, on sex work, but suffice to say here that the situation of Cambodia in the late 1990s does bear some relevance to understanding many of the current challenges facing the women, men, and transgender women now at risk. We should be mindful that the period covered here was, as hindsight has shown, the height of the AIDS crisis in the country. That time, thankfully, has passed.

What have proven much more resistant to change are Cambodia's political and human rights challenges. Hun Sen rules an authoritarian and deeply corrupt state which has delivered little for the impoverished majority of the population. The legacy of the countries' harsh past lives on in reports of regular beatings and torture in detention, in police and military impunity for these and other crimes, in the weak and politically controlled courts. The Khmer people deserve better. Perhaps their successes in responding to HIV are evidence of what they can achieve when given the chance – and the precious resources – to make a difference.

> To make peace we must remove the landmines in our own hearts which keep us from making peace: hatred, greed and delusion.
> (Venerable Maha Ghosananda)

Phnom Penh, the Cambodian capital city, has seen more than its share of suffering in recent decades. It was bursting with refugees during the Vietnam war, then abruptly emptied of its citizens at the start of 'year zero' by Pol Pot in one of history's most fanatical and destructive social 'experiments'. It has been invaded and occupied by the army of Vietnam. Then, when the international community marched in, the battered city on the Mekong was, for a time, the center of one of the United Nations' most ambitious missions. Elections followed which produced something like peace after a bloody electoral process.[2] But the elections failed to end the Khmer Rouge (KR) insurgency and left the country with a clumsy and ambiguous coalition government, two (incompatible) prime ministers, and a sporadically paid national army composed of several factions previously at war and still far from cohesive.[3] A violent and corrupt factionalism, scourge of past Khmer regimes, hobbled the fledgling administration. A future of authoritarian dictatorship looked tragically more likely in this transitional period than the growth of a living democracy, the return of the rule of law. And this is precisely what happened – Hun Sen did seize power in the 1997 coup, an infamous event known as the 'day of the grenades', and he has been in power since.

1996

Phnom Penh *circa* 1996 is a *non sequitur*. Coming by land, as I did from Ho Chi Minh City, is jolting, a mismatch of countryside and capital that makes sense only if you keep the recent past of this pained and ravaged place in mind. Once you cross the border at Moc Bai, at Cambodia's eastern end, you enter a landscape almost empty of people. It is pancake flat, the horizon broken only by the shaggy crests of sugar palms. The fields, or what used to be fields, are eerily empty, faintly marked squares of dust. The road from Ho Chi Minh to Phnom Penh, once one of the most dangerous on earth, has yet to be repaired. It is still not safe after nightfall, prone to banditry, Khmer Rouge (KR) attacks, or attacks by others (the police and the national army are frequently mentioned) often blamed on the KR. The hinterlands are heavily mined. What is most striking, especially after the bustling, intensively farmed Mekong Delta you leave behind, is the lack of human activity. There seems to be literally nothing happening: no farming, no trading, no mine sweeping, almost no traffic. The heat, dust, and silence don't give an air of peace; this is the silence of mass graves, of missing villages, of farms abandoned, of life stopped cold.

After a full day's drive through this landscape, arriving in Phnom Penh is like coming upon an Asian Las Vegas. The re-inhabited city is garish, gaudy, raucous, and thick with traffic. It is as though every car in the country, every building above two stories, every fast food outlet, every bank were in this city. And there *is*, absurdly, an immense new casino on the riverbank, dwarfing the worn Khmer and French buildings around it. Equally bizarre is a massive floating luxury hotel moored at the same bank. Downtown Phnom Penh has a booming red light district, spotted with brothels large and small, with Karaoke lounges and sleazy hotels, beer halls, and bars. It quickly becomes clear where the United Nations' billions were spent, and on what. Only pennies seem to have reached beyond the city limits. It's a despairing outcome to Cambodia's torment; crass luxury rising from the ashes. And more ashes for the poor. It is hard to argue that what Cambodia needed to rebuild after her trials was a casino, and not, say, a new university, a hospital, or some schools. Within an hour of arriving, I found myself longing for the country side again, for that terrain of emptiness and sugar palms where the difficulties of life were at least not covered with neon and tinsel. Cambodia now is not 'news'; the UN has moved on to other crises; the fortune spent here is unlikely to come again.

Information is hard to come by in post-election Cambodia. Journalists are favorite targets of the new death squads.[4] The man who appears to have taken control of the military and the police, and hence of the state, Second Prime Minister Hun Sen, does not tolerate criticism. His critics have a way of disappearing. Medical information is also scarce. Something like eight or nine Cambodian physicians survived Pol Pot's pogroms. There are almost no professors of medicine left to teach new ones. Health care in Cambodia is, by necessity, an affair of NGOs, relief agencies, foreign donors, and the UN. What scant information there is suggests grave problems, some only to be expected in the aftermath of longstanding social disruption, others perhaps unique to the agony of Cambodia.

As in the neighboring countries, HIV came late to Cambodia. Epidemic spread probably started some time between 1988 and 1990. As in Thailand and Burma, the virus found its requirements more than amply met. The origins of an HIV outbreak are ever obscure (and may not be terribly important, once local transmission chains are established and spread is under way) and this holds true for the land of Angkor. The virus may have entered the country across the Thai border in Cambodia's far west, where soldiers from both countries frequent a zone of cheap brothels outside the reach of both the law and health authorities. It may have come by ship along the southern coast where Burmese, Thai, Vietnamese, and Khmer fishing crews work the dangerous, pirate-infested waters of the Gulf of Siam. This coast is dotted with small islands that serve as rest ports, fueling stations, and venues for R & R; the larger islands are also spotted with brothels. Many women from the 'boat people' era of Vietnam's diaspora work in these remote shacks. Without passports, legal status, or access to health care, they are about as vulnerable to HIV as a human being can be. Another possibility, to which we will return, is an introduction from farther afield: the 20,000 young men who served as peacekeepers in the forces of the United Nations Transitional Authority in Cambodia (UNTAC).

The Cambodian National AIDS Prevention Committee is, given its limited resources, an impressive group. It is chaired by Ieng Sery Phan, a Khmer social activist, who has also long run the Cambodian Women's Development Association. She is a dynamic leader and has been able to garner enough donor support to begin to measure the spread of HIV and to focus on cleaning up the blood supply, at least in Phnom Penh. The committee estimated that in 1995 there were between 50,000 and 90,000 people in Cambodia with HIV infection, or roughly 2 percent of Cambodian adults. This is a serious problem, but it is the startling speed with which this population density has been reached that is more troubling. The prevalence of HIV among healthy young men donating blood in Phnom Penh went from 0.076 percent in 1991, or less than one in 1,000 men, to 3.62

percent in 1994, about one in 30. That is about as fast as a virus with HIV's infectiousness can spread, and suggests an epidemic out of control. These numbers, some of the only reliable data available on Cambodia, point to disaster.

Volunteer blood donors are an important 'marker' population. They are generally healthy young adults, as opposed to members of high-risk groups, and are usually persons selected to be at particularly low risk of having blood-borne infections like hepatitis B, malaria, HIV, or syphilis. Rates of any such illness in healthy people donating blood are more representative, and more generalizable, as regards what may be happening in the overall adult population of a city or country, than, say, rates among sex workers, or prison inmates. If we look at people from 'high-risk groups', the numbers are much higher than the blood donors. More than half of all sex workers in Phnom Penh were infected by 1995, up to one in ten police officers, perhaps one-third of soldiers along the Cambodian–Thai border, the wild west zone where cheap and unsafe brothels string the border like so many checkpoints. These very high rates are the stuff of headlines and they are disturbing, but the rate among blood donors means danger for many more people.

Cambodia today is not a society with the people or resources to deal with this kind of crisis, particularly as the effects of HIV spread will not be seen for several more years. The majority of recently infected blood donors are likely to feel quite well, and to be dealing with an array of pressing short-term problems: food, housing, security, rebuilding a life out of the ashes of the past, pushing, if they have the courage, for the return of civil society.

What seems clear from the information on soldiers, sex workers, and young men donating blood is that HIV in Cambodia is largely due to sexual transmission. While drug use is not uncommon, it is largely restricted to smoking the potent local marijuana, smuggled amphetamines, some opium smoking, and alcohol. The country is becoming a major marijuana exporter, and the drug is openly for sale in the old Russian Market, but injecting drug use seems to be rare.

Iatrogenic spread (that caused by unsafe medical practices) through blood transfusions and surgical procedures may be a bigger worry than drug use, although, again, the data are poor and scanty. We know that blood is screened for HIV in the capital, but the provinces and war zones are another matter entirely. These remoter areas are zones of emergency surgery and transfusions, thanks to that most destructive of weapons, the landmine. Getting information from these places can be life-threatening. One of the Khmer Rouge desta-bilization tactics is to kidnap and murder journalists, aid workers, and foreigners in general.

And then there is the war. Despite one of the largest UN efforts ever undertaken, and considerable international donor and NGO support, Cambodia is still fighting. The Vietnamese defeat of Pol Pot in 1978 generated a Khmer Rouge insurgency which has continued to threaten Cambodian governments ever since. Currently, more than two-thirds of government revenues continue to be spent on the war, draining the country of what limited funds are available for reconstruction. It is a hugely complex and protracted struggle, and the original Khmer Rouge leadership still runs it. Imagine a quarter of Germany under Nazi control 18 years after the Second World War, and still under the men who orchestrated the final solution.[5]

Cambodia is one of the most deeply wounded places on earth. You can see this on the face of anyone over 30. Much of the adult population suffers from post-traumatic stress syndrome (PTSS). An American friend, a psychologist working in Battambang, western Cambodia, from 1993 to 1995, told me that virtually everyone he knew exhibited at least some of the symptoms: recurrent night-mares, anxiety and panic attacks, flashbacks, irrational and extreme responses to memory 'triggers' of past horrors, substance abuse, depression, suicidal thinking, suicidal acts, rage. One of the most compelling symptoms of this national psychic wound was the well-described epidemic of blindness among older Cambodian women living in the U.S. in the 1980s. There were several hundred cases of this perplexing phenomenon, near or total blindness among seemingly healthy women of Cambodian origin. Several hypoth-eses were investigated, but the great majority of cases turned out to be psychogenic blindness, blindness born in the mind. These were women who had seen too much.

Many thousands of Cambodians were Khmer Rouge cadres, and thousands more have now grown up under the tutelage of men like Pol Pot and Ieng Sary, spending essentially their entire lives in the movement. Many have defected to the government side over time; the Khmer Rouge is thought to be down to less than 15,000 men in arms. But many, many more have served at one time or another, killing, raping, and torturing on command, often while still children themselves. National reconciliation in this tragedy means that these men and women will have to find a way to live again in the society they ravaged, that victims and torturers will have to pass each other on the street and not draw arms. Somehow the psychological scars of both sides will have to be healed.

It is a daunting prospect. Cambodia is awash with guns. Violence is used to settle even minor disputes. My psychologist friend in Battambang came closest to death not while the provincial city was under threat from the KR, but at a New Year's party. The next door neighbor thought the music too loud, and opened fire with a semi-automatic, killing the host. The thread that makes taking a human life difficult or impossible has been broken in Cambodia. The kind of scars that people here bear, and bury, have deep and powerful connections to the spread of AIDS, though these relationships are tangled, internal, difficult to investigate or illuminate. As Cambodia haltingly attempts to reconstitute itself, human rights abuses have continued, the use of force has not declined, the respect for individuals that marks civil culture continues to be undermined by the state. What is the nexus of these interwoven strands, a connection point between HIV and the internal nightmares of the Khmers? The sex trade is surely one.

Human rights and sex work   Trafficking of Khmer women and girls into the burgeoning sex trade has been increasing rapidly. HIV rates among these women are as disturbingly high as those in parts of Thailand, but HIV awareness, access to medical care, and condom use are all much less common. The use of force against these women includes not only forced prostitution, but beatings, rape, kidnapping, slavery, and murder. Contrary to the widely held belief in the power of economic progress to improve such conditions, these abuses are sharply on the rise in the new Cambodia. The Cambodian Human Rights Task Force, an indigenous NGO that is struggling to get the new government involved in halting these abuses, has collected and documented a heartbreaking array of cases. In March 1996, a fire in the red light district of Phnom Penh claimed the lives of two young Khmer women. Investigations by the Task Force later revealed that the women had been locked in their rooms and could not escape the blaze. NGO workers interviewed survivors from the brothel fire who alleged that the girls were under lock and key because they'd been recently trafficked against their will, and had refused to have sex with clients despite repeated beatings.

The Task Force has investigated other cases as well: in January 1996 in Battambang Province, a 13-year-old girl was beaten to death by a brothel manager who had bought her for prostitution. She also had refused to become a sex worker, despite repeated and worsening beatings, the last one being fatal. This girl's story came to light only because other girls enslaved by the same owner were so proud of her refusal to submit to rape. One managed to escape, and carried this tale of martyrdom to a teacher, who contacted the Task Force. The owner paid his way out of a trial. Another young woman forced into sex work died in a brothel fire in February 1996; she had been shackled to a bed in the brothel to prevent escape. These incidents are seen by NGO workers as part of a new trend in the sex trade: kidnapping and forced sex work by organized rings trying to cash in on the growing sex industry. The Khmer Rouge enslaved and killed for ideological, if insane, reasons. Sex slavery in the new regime is strictly a for-profit enterprise, but the methods are no less brutal, and the outcome no less horrific. It is perhaps a continuum, and it's not hard to imagine that some of the same people are involved. Was the brothel owner who beat a brave 13-year-old to death a Khmer Rouge torturer, or a brutalized victim himself? Almost everyone in this society was one or the other. Neutrality was not an option.

Phnom Penh is becoming a busy place for Asia's businessmen. This is another country, like Burma, where a significant chunk of investment is from the newly rich Pacific Rim states, and not the West. Japan, Thailand, Singapore, Malaysia, Taiwan, China, and Indonesia are all major players in the development business here. It is an open secret that many of these businessmen want sex when they travel. The rhetoric of 'Asian Values', or Confucian principles, falls flat if you take an evening stroll in Phnom Penh. The large and sleazy brothel district has signs not only in English and French, but in Chinese, Korean, Japanese, and Thai, offering 'full body massage', 'Karaoke with lovely hostess', a 'Good Time for You'.

The sex trade is not limited to the capital. Aid workers with the French medical charity Médecins Sans Frontières (MSF) working with women in the trade in the river port of Siem Riep, the gateway to Angkor, estimate that about 400 women are selling sex on any given day. (The overall population of the town is about 12,000.) Most of the business is local, according to MSF. The town is heavily militarized, and there are large demining teams, guards for the temple complexes, and many police. These men are poor and infrequently paid, but, thanks to the tourist and smuggling trades, there is some money in the local economy – enough to support a relatively large number of sex venues. Unlike Phnom Penh, where the trade is very much out in the open, Siem Riep is relatively discreet. If you're used to the way sex is sold in this region, it isn't hard to find, but the brothels don't line the main street. There are no real taxis in town, but local men sell rides on the back of their motorcycles. If you're a single man walking in town at night, these obliging fellows will immediately offer to take you to a girl. I never left my little guesthouse without attracting a steady stream of these motorized pimps.

The conditions in these upcountry brothels are abysmal. I spent an afternoon with Dr Else de Bruge, a Dutch MSF volunteer working with women and girls from Siem Riep's brothels. Her first challenge was education. The majority of her patients had almost no knowledge of sexually transmitted diseases, or of their own body parts. Condom use had become a huge issue for Dr de Bruge, and was much more complex than she had imagined. She had been at the job only a few months, and had begun thinking the issues were ones of availability, cost, and cultural appropriateness. She had found out quickly that condom use was very low or absent. But it soon became clear that many of the women, particularly the Khmer girls, were too traumatized to begin to deal with negotiating condom use with clients. They couldn't even bring themselves to discuss these issues with each other, with Else, much less with men. Brothel sex happens in silence, in the dark, and most of the men are drunk. Most of the young women had no choice but to accept clients who refused to use condoms, even men with STDs. Else began to rethink her approach, and spoke in terms of basic development, helping women to understand their bodies, to speak about sexuality, gradually to take some control of the lives they were now living. Dealing with protection, with 'safer sex practices' as we blandly call them, would follow later. While condoms are the cornerstone of prevention of sexual transmission, they have to be introduced into a context in which women who have never had to deal with sexual issues can begin to do this. It means touching condoms, looking at them, consciously thinking about being with men, and about their bodies. This is a painful, slow process, especially for women who are, to use a medical term, displacing themselves, going into psychological retreat from reality rather than face the drunk strangers already inside their bodies. We tend to be rather blithe about introducing condoms, and medical people are particularly bad about this, forgetting how difficult it is for most people to be rational and neutral about the body. Condoms go on an erect penis. Obvious enough. But for a village girl or a returning refugee, sold to a pimp and trafficked to a town far from home and family, even thinking about an erect penis is a nightmare. And you are asking her to learn how to put one on a man who is, in a very real sense, a part of serial rape. Many women do learn to do this, but more than half will become HIV-infected before they begin to protect themselves. Condoms are available in the markets in Phnom Penh, but are too expensive for many local people – prohibitively so for most in the countryside.

The International Red Cross is also active in Siem Riep. They have had to assist more than 38,000 returning refugees to the heavily mined province. (The country has had to contend with the return of nearly 400,000 refugees overall, many of whom have been unable to return to their homes due to fighting, landmines, or both.) In Siem Riep province, many of the returnees have become internally displaced persons, with fading hope of returning to their homes and past occupations. It takes little imagination to guess how vulnerable the women and girls of these families might be to brothel traffickers. A Red Cross officer in Siem Riep told me that HIV prevention is low on the list of priorities for the people of the province. He said this with great sadness; as a medical man, he knew only too well what was in store. He listed for me what he felt the priorities were in descending order of importance: finding enough food, securing housing, avoiding landmines, finding a job in the still marginal economy, and the end of the war. HIV prevention (buying condoms, for example) can indeed sound like a luxury, given this plethora of basic unmet needs. It is just this inability to respond to the seemingly distant and abstract threat of HIV when faced with more concrete threats to life that has led to the most severe HIV epidemics in Central Africa, where, in some countries, up to one-third of young adults may die. This may be where Cambodia is headed.

Official responses to the rise in the sex trade have so far been disturbing. In late 1995, three women employed in the sex industry were raped by uniformed police officers while taking an afternoon walk around Wat Phnom, an old temple at the northern end of the city. They were dragged into bushes near the temple and raped in daylight. The policemen's defense? 'Prostitutes cannot be raped because they are prostitutes.' The three women, with NGO support, pushed the new legal system for action. The officers were not tried, but were eventually fined token amounts. One of the people involved in helping the women raise funds for the trial told me that the most difficult problem was convincing the judges that a crime had been committed. The evidence for rape was overwhelming, but the judges agreed with the police that prostitutes 'couldn't be raped'. Judges, too, were targets of the Khmer Rouge, and most of the country's skilled jurists are long dead. Pressured to respond to the rising tide of rights abuses, deaths of prostitutes, and pressure from local and international organizations – particularly those that deal with child prostitution, such as End Child Prostitution in Asian Tourism (ECPAT) – the National Assembly began debating the issue in its 1996 legislative session. Rejecting calls for regulation of the sex industry, which had come from women's and health advocates, the legislators passed instead an order to 'eradicate' prostitution. (Eradication has unfortunate echoes in Cambodia.) Predictably, the order has had no visible effect on the sex trade, but it has made access to sex workers by their advocates more difficult and made the women even less likely to seek medical care.

A double lethality   Cambodia has another daunting challenge to face in HIV control: the small, cheap weapon that America, Italy, and China continue to produce to such profit, the landmine. The Land-Mines Advisory Group, a Phnom Penh-based organization struggling to deal with the problem, estimates that between 6 and 10 million landmines remain active in Cambodia, making it, with Angola and Afghanistan, one of the most heavily mined places on earth. Mine-clearing operations have been underway since 1991 and, given the difficulty of mine detection and de-activation, progress has been considerable. The Advisory Group reports that about 40,000 mines have been cleared since the operations began. At the current rate of 10,000 mines per year, it would take until late in the twenty-first century before Cambodia was safe for farming again, if no new mines were laid. The current rate of landmine maimings and killings is approximately 400 per month. Many of these injuries and deaths happen to children, who are among the most likely to wander off roads and beaten paths, to play in fields and forests.

Men of the UN   Cambodia offers some painful truths, if we would listen. We can learn of the legacy of American bombing, of Nixon and Kissinger's secret war, the depth that a human being can be brought to if pushed early and hard enough, the speed with which a nation can be destroyed and the agonizingly slow process of rebuilding one, and what can happen when HIV enters a ravaged society. For the international community, there is another dark teaching with wide implications. There is considerable evidence that the HIV epidemic in Cambodia was heavily influenced by the presence of UNTAC. The UNTAC mission was the first of its kind, and to date the only time the UN has actually served as the governing body for a sovereign state. It brought more than 20,000 people from numerous countries, including soldiers from the U.S., Western Europe, Bulgaria, Uruguay, India, Pakistan, Bangladesh, Thailand, Indonesia, Korea, and several African states. The great majority were young men, often of limited education. They walked into a country long closed to the outside world, starved for cash, and full of people eager to take their dollars. Prostitution was a likely outcome of this mix. It should have been just as likely that these troops were prepared to deal with HIV and other sexually transmitted diseases, but it didn't happen that way.

Local authorities are quick to blame UNTAC for the spread of HIV in Cambodia, insisting that prostitution was rare before the soldiers came, and HIV unheard of. This is taken as gospel in Phnom Penh's expatriate community, where tales of Bulgarian gang rapes and Uruguayan orgies with Khmer and Vietnamese girls are standard party fare. This is no doubt an over-simplification. But there is some evidence that the large number of international peacekeeping forces dramatically increased the demand for sex services. The infusion of cash from these forces into local economies after years of poverty and isolation was undoubtedly too great an attraction for many women (and brothel owners, managers, and traffickers) to resist. NGOs who were active with women in the sex trade before and during the UNTAC period report that sex workers, on average, doubled their nightly number of customers, from five to ten, during the UN mission.[6] Trafficking increased, as did migration of unforced professional sex workers from Vietnam.

The rates of HIV among blood donors in Phnom Penh also show that the 1991–1995 period was marked by explosive spread of HIV in the general population. This was the UNTAC era. Whatever else we can say about the relationships between the HIV outbreak and the presence of the UN forces, they were happening at the same time and in the same place, and to the same people; ordinary Khmers caught again in crossfire.

Soldiers from some of these countries undoubtedly came to Cambodia with HIV infection. Some may have been given HIV/AIDS education and condoms; other countries prohibit such education for soldiers, reasoning (there is no evidence for this) that such education might promote sexual activity. Muslim nations, like Pakistan, are notorious for these omissions. Other sexually conservative countries, like India, also resist such prevention activities. In either case, we do know that many of these soldiers left Cambodia with HIV infection. Studies of returning UNTAC soldiers in Uruguay and the U.S. have shown that most were infected with subtype E of HIV, which has previously been found only in Southeast Asia and Central Africa. They are likely to have become infected either in Cambodia or during visits to neighboring countries. Fully 15 percent of the Indian soldiers who served in UNTAC came home with HIV infection. This is an issue of more than academic interest. There is some evidence that subtype E may be more infectious through sex, and from female to male, than other subtypes. If subtype E has caused explosive heterosexual epidemics because it is more infectious through this route, then the global dispersion of subtype E from Cambodia is a potential public health disaster. It is a possibility that heterosexual epidemics in the West, long promised but in truth largely unseen, may now begin. It would be a tragedy indeed if peacekeeping missions, which the world supports for compassionate reasons, led to such suffering.

If there is any responsibility to be ascribed for this situation, it must lie with those governments which resist HIV-prevention programs for troops sent overseas. It is vital that future international efforts at peacekeeping, especially those of the UN, adopt comprehensive and frank HIV-prevention programs before such missions are undertaken. But the political feasibility of such programs is dubious, however important the consequences of not doing so. Failure to do what is needed on the part of the UN and its member states could make UN forces unnecessarily vulnerable to HIV infection as well as potential agents of HIV spread worldwide. Certainly, the outcome for the Khmer people has been a disaster. Khmer culture generally does not accept women who have been sex workers back into society. The large number of women who entered the trade during UNTAC now have few options but to continue. With Asian business activities increasing in Cambodia, the next wave of clients has arrived to replace the soldiers. Prostitution is likely to be further entrenched.

One step at a time Are there reasons for optimism in Cambodia? For hope? You find yourself asking this question almost daily in Cambodia. The kindness and sincerity of the Khmer people, despite the litany of challenges and abuses they have known, demands that you address it. While there is hunger in the country today, for food and for education, the Khmers I met hungered most for peace and for contacts with the outside world. Everyone I contacted for information and insight into the HIV situation responded quickly and positively, though many had cause to be afraid of doing so. This is a country where truth now matters intensely to people and they are eager to tell their stories. Conversations are long, food and drink and consideration are shared in abundance, criticism of the government is not held back. That generosity and courage could survive among so many people after what they'd known is more than inspiring. You come quickly to love the Khmer people for their tenacious belief in the goodness of other human beings. The young generation of Khmers who were children during, or were born after, the Pol Pot period are an impressive group. Walking the city, sitting in a tea shop, visiting a hospital or a school, you invariably end up in a conversation with these young Khmers. They want to practice English, but they are even more eager to talk about the future of Cambodia, their own futures and dreams. They are eager to learn, to travel, to help their country. While their concepts of democracy may be somewhat naive, democracy is the word that comes up again and again. Like the Chinese students of the 1989 democracy movement, what they want is a say in their own future, and what they are most against is the corruption of the elite. The nationalist rhetoric of the new regime is not fooling these young people. They know the real issue for most in power is personal profit. They want change. The country desperately needs reform, and it is these young people, not the UN, who will have to help bring it about. One only prays they can. They have at least one powerful example to follow.

The Supreme Patriarch of Cambodia, the Venerable Maha Ghosananda, is head of the kingdom's Buddhist clergy. He is one of the national figures at the center of Cambodia's revival of civil culture. Maha Ghosananda is a peace and democracy advocate, a social activist as well as a practicing monk and teacher of Buddhism. He is trying to bring about lasting national reconciliation through a revival of the spirit. His method is the Dhamma Yattra, the walk for peace. He has led six of these yearly mass pilgrimages thus far, going to every corner of the kingdom, bringing a message of *Mettha*, loving-kindness, to ravaged rural communities. The most recent Dhamma Yattra also carried an environmental message. Cambodia is being rapidly deforested. The marchers planted tree seedlings wherever they went.

Maha, as he prefers to be called by Western friends, is a man of 70, small and fit, his face a play of intelligence, compassion, and enthusiasm. I was granted an interview with him in Phnom Penh. I asked him first about reconciliation.

'I have offered the leaders of the Khmer Rouge, Pol Pot and his senior men, to ordain them as Buddhist monks. From our perspective, they have earned a large negative karma by causing so much suffering. Also, they are suffering themselves. They will have to begin to deal with this karma, either in this life or the next ones, so it is better for them if they start now. The sooner the better.'

'Did any accept the offer?'

'No. But they may someday. A good number of their soldiers are becoming monks. Many young men in Cambodia today are becoming monks, but I have to tell you that for most they choose ordination as a way of staying out of the army. They are not so serious about meditation. But it is still better than fighting. The *Sangha* is getting very big!'

'There is still so much violence and injustice in your country. And now AIDS has spread very quickly. I fear that the medical system will not be able to cope. How can your country be healed?'

'Suffering is a part of life. We are all suffering. But it is alright, it is improving, people are coming back to the temples, to the mosques, and beginning to practice mindfulness again, which is the only way to see through suffering. The government too, they will have to come around. And they will. Although suffering will continue. It always has.'

'When you led a peace march into the Khmer-Rouge-held territory, you and your followers were shelled. Are you worried about the next Dhamma Yattra?'

'We take one step at a time. One breath at a time. Keeping mindful of our actions, our minds. With each mindful step, we move closer to peace. This is the process and nothing can stop it.'

'I would like to come on your next march, but unfortunately I have to be back in Thailand.'

'Just take a few mindful steps with us, each day. It doesn't matter where you are. Khmer people are joining us in mindfulness in Thailand, in the States. You can do it in Chiang Mai. It doesn't matter.'

'Maha, tell me about Cambodian Buddhism. I've read that this is a Theravada country, but I see elements of Mahayana also. And much of Angkor was Hindu, wasn't it?'

'Yes, some of the people were Hindus. The names are not important, just the practice. In Cambodian Buddhism we have all three schools: Theravada, Mahayana, and Vajrayana. You will see some teachings, some texts, from all three. But the roots are the same. When we look around us at the world today, we see that the teachings are still very useful.'

'What about Buddhism in Cambodia today? You have lost so many monks and nuns.'

'We must take one step at a time, one breath at a time.'

Some Westerners find the teachings of Buddhism full of fatalism; the focus on suffering, and the acceptance of suffering, too passive or too likely to lead to tolerance of the intolerable. If you hear only the first (life is suffering) or second (the cause of suffering is attachment) of the four noble truths, this is understandable. But Buddhism goes two steps further. The third truth is the remedy for suffering (mindfulness, meditation, practice). And the fourth is of the reality of liberation. In a place like Cambodia today, in dealing with a social and medical disaster like AIDS, it is not hard to see suffering. What empowers and enlivens is being reminded by teachers like Maha Ghosananda that there is a way out.[7] The Buddha's last words say this with enlightened simplicity: *Work out your own salvation with diligence.*

Coda

In the past two decades Cambodia mounted a vigorous and largely successful fight against HIV. With donor support, and the vital technical and scientific input of the HIV community, the explosive outbreak of the 1990s was brought under control. The country and its leaders are proud of these efforts, and proud of the Millennium Development Goal award Cambodia received from the UN in 2010 for reducing HIV infections and achieving universal access to HIV treatment. The population, still poor, expanded from 9.7 million in 1992 to almost 15 million in 2012 – yet new infections declined 20 fold.

What does the future look like? External donor funds are declining – an outcome of success but also very much part of a wider trend in divestment from lower burden countries and a more focused effort on heavily burdened ones – a shift from Asia to Africa, where the needs are demonstrably greater. That leaves gay men, drug users, and the women Cambodia now prefers to call entertainment workers rather than sex workers more vulnerable – for they are facing ongoing spread of HIV in a country moving closer to declaring victory over the virus. Rates in gay men are increasing in 2016, albeit at much lower rates than in Thailand or China, but still a cause of real concern.

And Hun Sen? He is only 64, young by current dictatorial standards (Mugabe of Zimbabwe is 92, Museveni of Uganda, 72, Than Shwe of Myanmar, 83), and continues to hold Cambodian political life in his hands. This makes the plaudits he gets for Cambodia's AIDS successes a bit stomach churning. The West largely paid for the effort, Hun Sen allowed us to do so – and it was the Khmer people who did the hard work, despite the weak and ineffectual civil service they had to contend with.

Maha Ghosananda, my beloved mentor, died in March 2007, in the U.S., of complications of Alzheimer's Disease. He was 78. He had been nominated for the Nobel Peace Prize three times for his work on reconciliation in Cambodia, and for his two other great efforts there, demining and reforestation. His passing was a teaching (everything about this gentle, tactically savvy sage was a teaching) in the fragility of our minds in our physical bodies. Consciousness is, after all, an outcome of the dazzlingly complex functions of the wet brain, an organ, subject to inevitable decay. That a man with his depth of mental practice and state of realization should succumb to this untreatable brain disease was profound for me. There is no escape from the body.

I saw him last at an inter-faith event at the National Cathedral in Washington D.C. honoring His Holiness the Dalai Lama, several years before his passing. He'd been left alone at the small private reception for His Holiness, a tiny figure wrapped in bright orange, humbly waiting for someone to approach. The tenderness was the same.

But let me end with a happier day. I was back in Cambodia in the late 1990s, taking two American friends up country. Maha invited me to join him for a day's excursion, being deliberately cryptic about where we were to go and for what purpose. There was no entourage, just the two of us in the back seat of his small sedan, a driver in the front. We spoke of many things. The Khmer Buddhist tradition, how the HIV work was going, the efforts to protect Cambodia's ancient forests. After about an hour's drive north of Phnom Penh we came to a large, dusty country market. Maha excused himself and went off to shop. He and the driver returned with several big cages full of live monkeys, macaques, which they proceeded to strap into the now open trunk of the car. Loaded up with monkeys, we continued north. I said nothing, since he still seemed reluctant to speak. But he did volunteer that the monkeys were Cambodians, and they were due to be sold to Vietnamese traders. 'They eat them. We don't.'

North of the old city of Udong, we slowed in front of a large and enthusiastic crowd. Maha lit up, urging the driver forward and eager to get out of the car. As he stepped out the crowd parted and a beautiful ceremonial gold parasol was brought forward to escort him forward. Off he went, in grand state, to what looked a large, half-built structure. The monkeys were whisked off by some men and I was left alone to enjoy the scene. With no one to speak English to, I wandered, but was soon surrounded by a group of about 20 of the men. They were all dressed in loose white cottons, and wore either turbans or skull caps, so Muslims, not Buddhists. They were dark-skinned people for Khmers and looked like no one I'd seen in Cambodia or Thailand (or Laos and Vietnam for that matter.) One angular dark man with a handful of English words stepped forward with a huge smile and said, very loudly, 'You, which country?' 'Ah, America. We are Champa!' As he said this, still smiling, he gestured to the whole of the crowd, then hit his fist hard against his chest

So that's who they were. The Cham Muslims were the most persecuted of all Cambodia's minorities in the genocide. The survivors of the fall of the Kingdom of Champa to the Vietnamese 200 years before, close to half the Champa ethnic group had been murdered. They had no surviving Imam to consecrate their new Mosque. And so Maha, in his role as Supreme Patriarch, had agreed to serve. I never got near him again till the ride home, during which he happily explained how important it was for these people to have a mosque. Then I had to ask about the monkeys. 'All Cambodian religious buildings have monkeys – we feel they are not really alive without them. The ones here all died in the war times so we brought these to consecrate the temple. The Cham headman said he would protect them.'

A Buddhist Monk, consecrating a Mosque, with rescued monkeys, for a people who'd come close to eradication. That was the magic of Maha. In his *New York Times* obit one of his longtime students quoted him: 'We must find the courage to leave our temples and enter the temples of human experience.'

5 | LAOS: TRAVELS IN THE COLD WAR

Laos in 2016 remains a unique country. Almost alone in a densely populated and rapidly industrializing region, this is still a sparsely populated, largely rural place of green mountains, paddy fields, and a few modest sized towns and cities. Travelers have discovered Laos, it's lovely temples, beautiful landscapes, still cheap guesthouses and delicious, fiery food. But Vientiane and Luang Prabang maintain their leisurely pace – in striking contrast to the packed and charged megacities of the region, Bangkok, Ho Chih Minh, even Yangon in her rapid catch-up development hustle. The good news is that while Laos has an array of serious health problems, from water-borne illnesses and malaria to village fires and unexploded ordinance injuries, HIV is not a major contributor to Lao morbidity or mortality. The HIV rate is estimated at 0.2 percent of adults, or about 9,000 people living with the virus, even lower if we accept the Global Burden of Disease Study HIV estimates of 2015, which are closer to 7,000 infections nationwide, albeit with a very wide range (1,700 to 23,500 – an outcome of the uncertainty of the surveillance data). This is heartening and entirely not unexpected. The rural and lightly peopled mountains of Laos, the subsistence farming lives of most of her people, have likely not allowed for the kind of networks through which HIV most rapidly spreads. Having had such small numbers of people who injected drugs likely played a role too, though it is always tricky to posit what has or has not been determinative when an epidemic doesn't take off – or hasn't yet – in a given population. This is one of the reasons prevention impacts are so challenging to measure and attributions of success so fraught.

Lao gay men, bisexually active men, transgender women (here, as in Thailand, called *katoey*) and women selling sex all share higher rates of infection than the very low burden in most Lao men and women – but still at significantly lower levels than anywhere else in the region.

We brought Laos into our Hopkins Fogarty training program in 2001 as a partner with our many-year collaborative program with Chiang Mai University. For the next five years we conducted a number of HIV trainings in Laos, brought Lao colleagues to Chiang Mai and to Hopkins, helped establish their bioethics review committee. We did this working most closely with the Lao National Committee for the Control of AIDS, the NCCA, and its then leader, Dr Chansy Phimphachanh. Dr Chansy was a terrific partner. A warm and witty lady of great energy, she managed the delicate task of working with impatient donors, limited resources, and the cautious and bureaucratic Lao state. As we got to know each other better, she taught me a great deal about the workings of Lao and about how hard professionals in such constrained circumstances have to work to be effective. Her official salary, she once shared, was less than $40 dollars per month, the doctors on her team started at about $24 dollars.

Our Fogarty collaboration called for visits to some of the most remote and impoverished parts of Laos, the districts along the Myanmar (Shan State) and China–Lao borders. These areas were slated for road and bridge construction and other development projects. The fragility of the rural Lao in these areas was striking. Tribal people in threadbare clothes staring at Chinese market goods they couldn't afford – or trying to sell their gathered forest goods, mushrooms and greens, scavenged firewood, at the margins of the busy stalls.

Prosperity has not come to the people of Lao – nor has political change. She is still ruled by a communist party, the Lao People's Revolutionary Party, who came to power after the U.S. defeat in Vietnam in 1975. Tight control of information and suppression of dissent are still the leadership's stock in trade. The fate of one prominent rights activist, Sombath Somphone, who was abducted by men in plainclothes during a traffic stop in Vientiane in 2012, remains unknown. If he is in prison or detained by the authorities, he is likely sharing in the same very harsh conditions in which other political prisoners have been held; in chains or manacles, unlit cells, or in solitary confinement, all of which have been credibly reported by survivors.

1996

The health status of the people of Laos remains poorly documented and little studied. There is little on Laos in the medical literature, and the Lao lay media are limited and heavily censored. Government publications are fairly crude propaganda and of uncertain credibility. Many rural areas remain beyond the reach of researchers and the press, and in some areas even of the government. There are few roads, and there has never been a yard of rail. After the region-wide floods of 1994 there were persistent rumors of severe rice shortages, even of famine, in several parts of Laos; these reports were neither confirmed nor denied. In 1995 there were reports of a major outbreak of cholera in several flooded provinces; these reports also were neither confirmed nor denied. Parts of Laos are so uncharted that in 1995 a new ethnic group was discovered in the mountains, a people who had managed to miss both the French colonial period and the nine-year war with the Americans. Laos is not on the information highway. It is a place to which you have to *go*.

One large survey of HIV was reported from Laos in 1994. This was a study among 9,449 persons resident in Vientiane, the capital, between January 1990 and April 1993. The survey was a collaboration between the Hôpital Mahosot, Vientiane, and the Hôpital Cochin, Paris. They found only a few cases: 18 were confirmed out of the whole sample, about 0.2 percent, roughly one in 500 persons. The majority of infected persons, 13 of the 18, were women aged 15–29. Twelve of these young women had worked as sex workers in either China or Thailand prior to testing HIV-positive. Most of the tests (5,176) done in this survey were among blood donors. Tellingly, none were HIV-infected (95 percent of these donors were men.)

Based on this evidence, if we take it as reliable, we could say several things about HIV in the Lao PDR in 1993. Compared to its neighbors (Laos has borders with Thailand, Burma, Cambodia, Vietnam, and China) there wasn't much. The finding in blood donors is encouraging; this is a large sample and it suggests little spread in the general population. What HIV cases there were turned up among Lao women and girls who had worked in neighboring countries' sex industries; these were more likely to have been imported cases than evidence of local spread.

But there were some problems with these findings. Vientiane is not Laos. This was an urban sample in an overwhelmingly rural country. The introduction to the Mahosot–Cochin study bears some scrutiny.

HIV infection in Lao Republic

B.C. Prasongsith, P. Blanche, K. Phouvang, S. Insisiengmay,
V Rajpho, D. Sicard.

A rising incidence of human immunodeficiency virus (HIV)
infection has been reported in Thailand and to a lesser extent
in Southern China. The Lao People's Democratic Republic
(Lao PDR) is located in the heart of the Indochinese peninsula,
between Burma and China to the north, Cambodia to the south,
Vietnam to the east, and Thailand to the west. The opening of
the Lao economy, the building of routes and the completion of
the Mekong River bridge between Thailand and Lao PDR
could lead to an increase in the incidence of HIV infection. Lao
PDR is 80% mountainous, with a low density of population
($17/km^2$), mostly rural, so that a national sero-survey is difficult
to organize.

This introduction nicely shaped what could be called the Lao dilemma.
The heart of Indochina is land-locked, sparsely populated and poor.
But it is surrounded by crowded countries in dynamic periods of
growth and change, with booming economies and increasingly
serious social problems. Laos's neighbors want Laos open. They
want hydroelectric power from its mountain rivers, they want its
timber, they want trade on the Mekong River and they want roads.
As it stands, Laos's continued self-imposed isolation blocks road or
rail connections between Thailand and China, between Thailand
and Vietnam, and between northern Thailand, northwestern Laos,
the Shan states of Burma, and Yunnan, the 'Golden Quadrangle'
economic and travel zone that all the other countries agree could
make them richer if Laos would only comply. So far, the Party has
resisted.

The Thai–Lao Friendship Bridge mentioned by the Mahosot–
Cochin researchers was built with Australian development funds. It
officially opened in 1994, connecting Vientiane with Nong Khai, in
Thailand's northeast. Ordinary Laotians were not allowed to cross
it without special permission, because of government concerns over
'traffic safety'. Once across, they were usually allowed only three
days in Thailand, and are not allowed to leave Nong Khai province.

HIV is just one of a list of threats that Laotians perceive will come
with openness and travel. The Party, a Lao contact suggested, is

more afraid of ideas and information than viruses. The leadership may have other worries as well. Increasing openness might reveal the extent to which their oligarchy is supported by opium revenues. Laos is number three, after Afghanistan and then Burma, in Asia's opium and heroin production. Not surprisingly, the Lao PDR was the first government in the world to recognize the SLORC, three weeks after the 1988 crackdown in Burma. Ties are close. Heroin was, with hydroelectric power, timber, and a small coffee crop, the only significant foreign income earner the country had.

The heroin business also involved the Lao leadership's unresolved conflicts with the nation's traditional opium growers, the Hmong and Yao ethnic nationalities. These peoples began opium cultivation to pay the head tax demanded by France during the colonial period. They fought for the French, and subsequently the Americans, during the Indochinese wars; these loyalties led to severe reprisals by the communists once they took power. Some estimates are that a quarter of the Hmong population, some 250,000 people, were killed, and another 200,000 driven into exile, by the Pathet Lao. Many of these refugees found shelter in Thailand and, eventually, in the U.S. Those that did not make it out of the Thai refugee camps were still there in 1993. The repatriation of these remaining Hmong refugees back to Laos is one of the last acts of the Vietnam-era passion play. It was almost completed in 1996, but tensions still ran high. There were rumors of a resurgent Hmong resistance to the Lao regime, rumors that again have been difficult to verify or discount. What was happening in the highlands was as hidden as the roadless ranges themselves.[1]

How vulnerable was Laos to HIV? Between 1994 and 1996 I made three trips there in an attempt to answer this question, to study this enigmatic place in the 'heart of Indochina'. The first was a short and unproductive trip to Vientiane. The second a longer journey, overland and by boat, down the Mekong to Luang Prabang, the old capital. The third, a visit to the most heavily bombarded place on earth, the Plain of Jars, and from there north, to poppy growing areas near the border with Vietnam, what used to be called the Ho Chi Minh trail.

Vientiane Arriving in Vientiane from Chiang Mai is like stepping off a flight from JFK into a wide Montana afternoon. The skies are astonishing. The afternoon I landed it was a high clear blue with puffy banks of cumulus overhead. There was a band of soft river light to the south, over the Mekong, vertical rain falling to the far north, a fierce brilliant sun just off-center to the west. Such skies are history in Chiang Mai, where bands the color of nicotine hang perennially over the valley, and even the bluest reaches are dull with dust and lead.

Vientiane is slow. What little traffic there is glides over the rutted roads with a cadence more like boating than driving. It's striking after frenetic Thai traffic. The population was supposed to be 493,505 in 1995, but it feels more like one-tenth of that. The city sits beside a wide stretch of the Mekong. Where the flood waters have receded, locals have planted vegetable patches in the river bed, giving the city a scraggy backdrop of corn tassels. The feel is much more of a provincial town than a city, a town with several grandiose monuments which suggest not so much that this is a capital city, but that the state they are meant to represent is something of a historical fiction, and an unconvincing one. There is the Lao version of the Arc de Triomphe, rising high above a traffic circle and facing the Presidential Palace in a dramatic layout that is pure Paris. Instead of power, it suggests a very threadbare colonial vision of what might have been.

The same can be said of the enormous and criminally ugly constructions of the Soviets. Peeling and cracking, they suggest less the fraternity of a socialist international than another vision of Laos which contrasts jarringly with the actual town, a place of low, ramshackle houses, banana trees growing out of pavements, kids and chickens and dogs padding about in the dust.

There is no daily newspaper, but the *Bangkok Post* is available intermittently. There is a weekly *Vientiane Times* in English, fascinating reading from a cultural, if not a news, standpoint. What educated Laotians actually use for news is a mimeographed daily 'fact sheet' which has telegraphic shorts on international matters extracted from the Chinese *Xinhua* news service, as well as bulletins from the Lao Government. It is actually written in decent English, and, surprisingly, reported news both of rice shortages in Luang Prabang province and of a cholera outbreak north of Vientiane.

I will spare you the frustrations of trying to arrange meetings in Vientiane. A low-level official chuckled at my attempts and told me that 'Lao PDR' stands for Laos Please Don't Rush. Expatriates have it as Lao Per Diem Required – if you don't pay officials to attend meetings, the doughnuts and coffee are all yours.

The one, not unqualified, success of this trip was a journey inland to one of the large dams built to harness Laos's hydroelectric power. We made the journey inland in a huge Chinese flatbed truck. This took us north of Vientiane and up toward the highlands. There were very few other vehicles on the road once we left the city (although we still managed to collide with one, a Soviet Laika sedan that our Chinese charger crunched with impunity). The only significant traffic was of logging trucks, a steady stream of them bearing the trunks of immense trees heading north to China, whose booming economy is starved for hardwoods, long a symbol of wealth to the Chinese. We never made it to the dam, as our vehicle lost several gears, and ceased to be able to negotiate the steeply graded roads. But we did get fairly far into the countryside, and it is here that the country reveals something more of itself.

Rural Laos is, if anything, slower than Vientiane. It is very much a traditional subsistence economy of small scattered towns and villages. There is little evidence of trade, or of any surpluses with which to trade. With the exception of saw mills cutting timber for the trucks, there is not much sign of anything like industry. Where the land is flat and has enough water, it is paddy country. But that year's monsoon had been heavy and much of the lowland was still flooded.

The countryside is an ethnic patchwork as complex as the paddy plots. Each village seems ethnically distinct from the next; beside a Hmong community is a Tai Dam one, then a Lao, then a Yao, then perhaps another Tai Dam, or subgroup of Laos. What they have in common is poverty. Most houses are simple shacks without running water or electricity. Toilets are outdoor latrines, often built over running streams. Where there are sewage systems (we saw a few in the larger towns) these are raw open drains. It's not hard to see why cholera remains such a problem here. The men thigh deep in the paddy are also vulnerable to the flukes and parasites so common in these regions. Children with kwashiorkor were common in some villages, especially the Hmong ones, where most of the younger kids we saw were malnourished.

Luang Prabang Luang Prabang is the old capital of Laos, the royal city of the Lao Kingdom in earlier times. It is on the Mekong, like Vientiane, but on a section of the river that cuts deep into the country, and is ringed by mountains. While no longer a commercial center, it retains its place as the gem of Lao culture and architecture. In Lao it's usually called Mong Luang, main city. To get there you can cross Thailand's far north by road, and cross the Mekong where it forms the Thai–Lao border. This takes you to Ban Huai Sai, where you can catch freight boats to Luang Prabang.

Ban Huai Sai looks modern and ugly, but is in fact an old trading town. It was here, in the eighteenth and nineteenth centuries, that trading caravans from Yunnan came down from the Silk Road and met the Mekong. They crossed with their goods to Chiang Khong in Thailand, and traded them in Chiang Rai and Chiang Mai. They then crossed back to take the river to the old Lao capital. This ancient route is catching on again. Chinese laborers come down to Ban Huai Sai looking for work in Laos. Goods come up from Chiang Rai, are ferried across, and go either north by road or down the Mekong. The goods include guns, which are sold openly on the streets of Ban Huai Sai, and the chemicals necessary to turn opium into heroin. North of Ban Huai Sai, it has been reported (but, of course, not confirmed) that there are several large heroin refineries. Shan opium is also reportedly refined in northern Laos. The old Silk Road takes the purified white powder to Kunming, in China. From there it is flown to Shanghai, then Hong Kong, then out to the markets of the West. So this small and seemingly sleepy little river port is one key link in the chain that eventually leads to the agonies of Harlem, Newark, and Watts.

The road north out of Ban Huai Sai, which connects Thailand to southern China, is slated to be a key part of the growth zone of the economic quadrangle. Its development is planned with support from the Asian Development Bank (ADB). If this comes to pass, Ban Huai Sai will change radically. How this will affect the heroin trade is yet another unknown. (The idea of the conservative ADB helping to improve the infrastructure for the heroin industry would be amusing if it were not so sad.)

Just after dawn, we climb onto the tin roof of a freight boat. We will sit on this roof for two days. Two days in which we see perhaps 20 villages altogether, one small market town, and miles and miles of dense green mountain forest.

Several of the villages we pass are Hmong. These are new villages, though because they're bamboo and thatch, they look as old as any of the other river-bank hamlets. This area is not traditional Hmong land. They were always mountain farmers, not riverfolk. But the deep mistrust of the Hmong for the government in power has kept them close to Thailand, where the refugee camps are only a few hours by boat. And, like the Khmer refugees, many Hmong cannot go home owing to landmines and unexploded 'ordnance'.

The river is swollen. I sit with the captain for a few hours to avoid the sun. We are carrying asbestos roof tiles to Luang Prabang, and the barge is overloaded. The wheel he turns is rigged to iron chains that run on each side of the 30-foot craft, and turn the rudder at its end. Because of the weight and length of the barge, he has to anticipate a wide backswing, and glide the boat over rapids as its stern trails now wide to the left, now too far to the right. The chains are responsive to the wheel, but the boat is not easily handled, and he is in constant motion, eyes on the rocks, the currents, the way ahead. In two days of constant travel he never comes close to a rock, never comes near a spill over the rapids, never slows down. Underdevelopment develops people, if nothing else.

The country is spectacular. The mountains are dense and closely packed, dropping steeply to the river with dark granite walls. Everything is green after the rains. There is very little sign of people here. Every few kilometers you see what looks like the remains of a field, some scattered plantings of corn or banana. In some stretches we move for several hours without seeing a soul.

When we stop for the night, the captain invites us to drink shots of the local moonshine, called Lao Lao. Made from rice, it has a faint taste of licorice, with a hint of gasoline. It comes in a plastic bag, and there is only one glass, filled to the brim and emptied in one fiery gulp. After the third, or fourth, I actually like it, though there is the lingering fear of it being methanol, not ethanol, and waking up permanently blind.

Sitting around the fire after dinner, I ask the men if they have heard of AIDS. Yes, they have, they know it's spread by sex, and they know it kills you, but they all agree that it is only in Thailand, not in Laos. I ask the captain if he thinks he is in any danger of becoming infected. 'No. Because I don't do anything that would put me in danger. I am married, I stay with my wife. She is very beautiful. And I don't go to brothels, even in Vientiane.'

Dawn, when it finally comes, is damp and chilly. Our captain is up before first light, working the fire. After a sickeningly sweet coffee each, we crawl back onto the boat and huddle on the wet tin roof. If it wasn't hard to get to this place, it wouldn't be what it is. All the comfortable places in this crowded region are packed to the gills.

Another day of green mountains, pink buffaloes, blue kingfishers, and the river twisting and winding its way through gorges, over rapids, into wider, slower stretches. We have cut sharply away from Thailand now; and the river is running almost due east toward the city. There are still only a handful of hamlets and fields cut out of hillsides. The buffaloes must be inbred: more than half are albinos, pink where caked mud has cracked on their hides, with milky white muzzles and dull gray eyes.

There is no sign as we approach that the old city is near. There are no outlying towns, no roads, only a few more long-nosed boats, and a handful of barges. The city doesn't actually appear as we come round the last bend. There are just banks coated with garbage, and four or five stairways leading up from the shore. Luang Prabang is a town of about 8,000 people.

In the afternoon we visit the house of a Lao family who sell old weaving and embroidery, one of the Lao high arts. The woman who runs the business is about 40, a classic beauty: delicate features, wide-set cocoa-brown eyes, and thick, straight black hair to her waist. Her mother joins us, an equally lovely old lady, with the same eyes, and her white locks in a high bun. They were connected to the court in the old days, and have suffered greatly. Their men are gone. Beside the cash register in the shophouse are several photos of their daughter in traditional dress. Another stunning face, and impossibly slender limbs and waist. The mother tells me proudly that her daughter was 'Miss New Year' in the last beauty pageant. A Thai businessman paid a 10,000-Baht bride-price for her and took her to live in Bangkok. They have not seen her since, but are sure that she is alright, for the Thai man was rich. The Thai man told the family that he wanted her for a wife, and I hope that is true, but the likelihood is that she is locked in a brothel or massage parlor somewhere, servicing an endless string of men. There are many versions of this story, and 10,000 Baht (about U.S.$400) is the standard rate for women trafficked into the flesh trade. Wives usually cost more.

The Luang Prabang Provincial Hospital is on the main street in town, ringed by a low stone wall, behind which is a lawn gone to seed. The buildings are single-story French, circa 1930s, and clearly not renovated since. Rather than go through official channels, which I've been told can take months, I tell a nurse crossing the grass that I need to see a doctor. She leads me into a large empty room, with one desk and two low benches in a corner. A young woman joins us after a few minutes, and this is the doctor. She has a bright open face and a welcoming smile. I give her my card, explain the purpose of my visit, and ask her if she has a few minutes to talk. She speaks Russian (trained in Moscow in Internal Medicine), Lao, a bit of French, and some Thai. I speak Thai, fair French, and understand about half of what is said in Lao. This leads to a word-salad conversation, a Tower of Babel for two, but, medicine being medicine, we can passably follow each other. She does not offer her name, or a card, and I sense that I shouldn't push for this.

The hospital has 200 beds, and a staff of 12 medical doctors supported by another 20 or so health aides and nurses. As Laos has no medical school, all the doctors have been trained overseas, the very elderly in France, but since the 1960s in the Soviet world: in the Soviet Union itself, in Cuba, Hungary, and Vietnam. Now that Soviet aid for education has stopped, they are hoping to send the next generation to Thailand, where there is no language barrier, and no long Russian winters.

The single largest problem here is malaria, which is endemic in much of Laos. More than half the in-patients are malaria cases, especially children with cerebral malaria. Many of the current cases have falciparum, the most aggressive of the four malaria parasites. Antibiotic resistance is a major problem. After malaria, tuberculosis is next, then diarrhea, cholera, malnutrition, and accidents, which often lead to infected wounds. As we walk the crowded, dirty wards, it is clear that HIV would be a disaster here. Because people with HIV infection are so susceptible to tuberculosis, and there is already so much TB, an African situation, with both diseases running rampant, could make this place a charnel house.

'Have you seen any HIV cases here? Any clinical AIDS?'

'We don't have resources to test as many people as we should. This we know. We test women from Luang Prabang coming home from working in Thailand, because we know many of them have worked in brothels there. So far we have found only three with HIV. They all came back with money and got married soon after, so we know HIV is here. We don't see many heroin addicts who use needles. Even we can't get enough needles! But I personally am worried because now we have so many Chinese laborers, and laborers coming in from the Shan states. Next year the government wants to have direct air flights from Chiang Mai to Luang Prabang, so we must be prepared. We are surrounded by AIDS countries.'

'Do you think the medical staff here would like to have some training in AIDS control and care?'

'Definitely, yes. There is a lot we don't know. But you will have to speak to the minister of health about this, in Vientiane. I will introduce you to his deputy in Luang Prabang.'

'What about prostitution here?'

'We don't really have that, only in Vientiane.'

'I was told there are prostitutes at the R hotel, and at the disco.'

'Yes, that is true.'

The head of the Pediatrics department, another woman, was trained in Havana. I dig up my high school Spanish from somewhere, and we are back to word salad, this time with a salsa twist. She shows me a ward full of children with cerebral malaria, a major cause of death here. There are two little boys, brothers, with their father and grandfather, both boys in deep coma after a three-day walk to the hospital. The men are anguished, startled to see a white face, and then hostile when it's clear that I have nothing to offer their dying sons.

The surgery is a part of medical history, with used surgical gloves washed and hung up to dry like hand towels. There is an autoclave, actually working, to sterilize the tools, a donation from the U.S. from before the fall of Saigon. The intensive care unit, such as it is, has no working oxygen, no suction, no ventilators. This is not a place to have a serious illness, and it is the only hospital for hundreds of miles in these rugged mountains.

'What do you do for cases that need oxygen?'

'We try to get them to Vientiane by plane. If they have money, and if we can arrange it, we send them to Udon.' Udon is the Air America base in northern Thailand from which we sent over the payloads dumped on these people for nine long years.

Altogether I talked with seven physicians, all women. I found out later that they each earn 38,000 Kyip a month, less than U.S.$40. The government prohibits doctors from having private clinics, which is why, I find out later, there are no men left working as physicians – you can't support a family on a physician's wages.

On our way to meet the deputy minister of health, we leave the hospital compound and walk to a small building next to a gas station. The walls are covered with health promotion posters, several of which I recognize as AIDS posters put out by the Thai authorities. A staffer tells us they are in Lao, but the writing is clearly Thai. They show bar-boys dancing in bikinis, and people with horrendous end-stage disease – useless messages here, where HIV will not spread though non-existent male hustlers, or wasted dying bodies, but through healthy looking young men and women, as it has throughout Asia.

'Good morning, I am the deputy here. Ah, you are from Thailand. Interested in AIDS, I see. Of course Thailand has a lot of AIDS. We don't have this problem here. There have been no cases of HIV or AIDS in Luang Prabang. Why not? Well you see, we do not have any drug users here, and we do not have prostitution. Also, Lao people are not involved in this homosexuality. So we really have no way for HIV to spread here.'

The young lady doctor spoke up, and I liked her hugely for her courage.

'We have had three cases already, sir.'

'Three, I thought it was only two. Yes, well, one has gone back to Thailand already for treatment.'

'We were hoping to do an HIV course for the medical staff here. Do you think the Ministry would support this idea?'

'Oh yes, why not, we are very open to improving our capabilities. Always open.'

'Could I ask you about drug use? Do you see this as a problem in Laos?'

'It is a problem in every country, isn't it? But it is much less common now than in the past. Our people are very simple, you understand. And we have taken steps.'

'Steps?'

'When the Americans were here, Laos was full of these drugs. Now you see, it is only some of the older people, tribal people.

They think of opium as a medicine. This is changing, but it is slow. Perhaps you should speak to my superior. He can tell you more.' And then, at last, a name: the minister of health for the Lao PDR, and his address. We are far from the communist mainstream here, but the archetype, the party functionary toeing the line, is alive and well in Luang Prabang.

The Plain of Jars   The Plain of Jars (Plain des Jarres – PDJ to war buffs) was one of the most heavily contested theaters of the secret war in Laos. The U.S. had no ground troops there, just CIA operatives and the Hmong. The North Vietnamese had perhaps 70,000 troops on the high plateaus around Xiang Khoang, the only major town on the PDJ. The U.S. strategy was to bombard the communists by air, waging an aerial campaign against the Ho Chi Minh trail without using U.S. ground troops. This went on for nine years and was a manifest failure. When the U.S. had had enough of bombing and went home, the Hmong were swiftly defeated, and the Plain of Jars fell under Vietnam's control. The people of Xiang Khoang had lost their city, their countryside, and, in many cases, their lives. The region today is desperately poor. The U.S. mission was in one sense a success: we wanted 'to bomb them into the stone age', and just about did.

There was no plane available on the day we wanted to go to the PDJ, but an old Soviet transport helicopter had been pulled out of storage from somewhere. The door didn't exactly shut, which meant the Lao flight attendant spent the entire ride holding on to it. The view of the mountains was especially nice through the seams in the chopper floor.

Once airborne you pass quickly out of the settled plain around Vientiane. For many miles there is nothing below but green mountains, snaky rivers cutting through unfarmed valley floors, and high stone ridges bare of trees. The country dries out as you head north; the forests are replaced first by low scrub, then by bare earth studded with rock. About 50 miles from the PDJ the craters begin to appear. It is impossible to see now what was being bombed. Many high brown ridges, completely devoid of green, are pocked and punched and bitten with craters. What had been there? Villages? Troops dug into bunkers? Cattle grazing? Were there forests? Was this landscape always lifeless, or did we do that? Nearer to Xiang

Khoang the craters are virtually everywhere. It looks like smallpox, on land instead of skin. There are huge circular chunks missing from the scattered fields, from the sides of hills, gouged out of the flat spaces. The old city of Xiang Khoang, capital of an ancient and little documented Lao–Thai kingdom, was bombed into oblivion. Erased. The new town, which we are just about to enter, looks bleak from the sky. Everything standing is post-1975. There is no evidence, from the air, of the famous jars.

After a soft slow landing we climb out of the helicopter into a blast of frigid, dusty wind. The plain around us is brown, bleak, empty, more like Mongolia than Southeast Asia. The arrivals building is a rattan-walled shack. We get our police stamp, and we meet Duang Sai Jai (in English 'to add stars to your heart'). He's a young Lao guide with a jeep and he speaks Thai. After a few minutes of negotiation, we're off.

Driving through this countryside is a lesson in the aftermath of war. The surviving people, in their poverty and ingenuity, have come up with an incredible array of uses for what gets left after nine years of bombardment. Their pig troughs are made of bomb casings; the rice barns are raised off the ground on bomb casings; a farmer's plough uses the base of a tank. Scrap from the war is used to make water pumps, fence posts, and shack foundations. In the end, what fell from the sky was made of metal. It is a pity we didn't just drop real pig troughs.

The jars of the PDJ are a fitting attraction for the place. Cut from solid stone, and varying in length from perhaps four to eight feet, they are, quite simply, giant stone jars. Their meaning is lost, and the culture that generated them is unknown (and given the destruction here is likely to remain so). They sit on the land with their open mouths saying whatever they were meant to say to an uncomprehending audience. So too the bomb craters. What was it for and why was it done? What do they mean now, to the local people? The population of Laos is exceptionally young, the older generation having been greatly reduced in number by years of war. The people of Xiang Khoang are mostly post-war kids. They want to learn English, wear blue jeans, dance in discos, and study abroad. The battles that cost their parents everything have been over for 20 years. Duang Sai Jai would like to go to university. Laos does not have a university. He would like to go to Bangkok (they have better brothels there than in Vientiane, he tells me). But it is 'difficult', he says, as he has no family connections to the leadership. The Party is not about to let Duang Sai Jai and his friends travel to the capitalist nation next door. And they are never going to forget the nine years of fire falling, day and night, from a faraway enemy in the skies.

We pass through the town of Ponsavanh on our way to the mountains. The modern town was built by the Soviets, after the U.S. destroyed the original one. The people walking along the cold, dusty road are about as poor as you can get; we pass several kids with the orange hair of kwashiorkor, little girls carrying enormous bushels of sticks, gaunt old men on Chinese bicycles, hatless and gloveless in the bitter air. We stop in the market to get some water for a three-hour drive north. There are some mealy cabbages and turnips, some wilted lettuces, and little else. One Khmu tribal woman is selling three freshly killed porcupines. She sits before the fat rodents laid out on a board, methodically plucking quills from their skins with a short knife. Another woman, a blue Hmong, has a pair of grey-green magpies for sale. They've been snared, and their beautiful plumage is intact. It is a species I have never seen before, with a long, curved vermilion bill, white eye patches, and the distinctive long banded tail feathers of the family. Alive, they would be worth a fortune, by Lao standards, on the illegal bird market. Here, they are being sold for meat.

There is only one road going north out of Ponsavanh. You could take it to China if there was a border crossing at its end, but apparently there isn't. The border with Vietnam is about 40 kilometers east of this road, which explains why it was bombed so thoroughly. The land is dry, rocky hills, too steep for rice, but perfect for poppies. Actually the flowers are not in bloom at this time of year; the plants are only about a foot high, and look more like a kind of spinach than those lovely red flowers that carpet the hillsides. The road north has many poppy patches, but Duang Sai Jai insists that the real fields are one ridge over from the road. The fields we do see are mostly tended by little girls. There is little to do but weed at this time of year. It looks like lonely work for children, and there seem to be no adults around, nor even any houses that these small laborers might go home to. I had expected something more sinister than this, but opium is a poor people's crop. The people who grow it see the least fraction of its profits. The money these little girls generate must run to many millions, but it gets laundered and invested in another world, and spent in yet another, the place where the bombs came from.

How vulnerable is Laos to an HIV epidemic in the future? As the sages say, it depends. After these journeys I'd come to think the politburo might be right to go slowly in terms of opening Laos to its neighbors, to trade, investment, and development. Laos was fragile, its economy marginal, its society still in tatters after years of war. Change would inevitably come to the heart of Indochina, but in what form and on whose terms? One question remains relevant: will HIV follow the new roads here, as it did into the hinterlands of Africa? It still easily could. Would development lead Laos out of the opium-growing business or push it further down a darker road? Time is still moving at the Laotians' chosen pace, but the neighbors are impatient.

6 | MALAYSIA: ETHNICITY, ACTIVISM, AND AIDS

Over period of 29 years, the country has observed tremendous biomedical and behavioral advances in the HIV prevention, diagnosis, and treatment. As a result, there has been a significant reduction of new cases by almost half from 28.4 per 100,000 population in 2002 to 11.7 cases per 100,000 population in 2014. Malaysia is a country with concentrated HIV epidemic with infection rates remains high above 5% among key populations (KPs) especially among PWID [people who inject drugs], female sex workers, transgender and men sex with men (MSM) population. By 2013, Malaysia has enjoyed almost 50% decline in new HIV cases since its peak in 2002 (6,978 cases). But in 2014, new cases has edged up from 3,393 in 2013 to 3,517 HIV. Malaysia is estimated to have about 91,848 people living with HIV (PLHIV) by end of 2014 ... In general, PLHIV in this country is predominately male (89%). As the epidemic spread, the pattern progressively shifted towards increasing infection rates in female with male/female ration from 9.6 [to 1] in 2000 to 4.5 in 2010 to 4.0 in 2015. (*Malaysia 2015: Country Responses to HIV/AIDS*, Ministry of Health, December, 2014)

Malaysia has had a remarkable response to HIV over the last two decades. Remarkable because the country was able to change direction away from one of the harshest anti-drug regimes in Asia to adoption of harm reduction as an approach, and needle and syringe exchange and methadone as pragmatic public policy. Sustained advocacy led to implementation of harm reduction in 2005. Declines in new HIV infections were seen quickly among Malaysia's large population of people who inject drugs (PWID). This effort was led by an unlikely heroine. Professor Adeeba Kamarulzaman is a soft-spoken, exquisitely polite physician, trained in infectious diseases in Australia. A Malay, a practicing Muslim, and a mother, Prof. Adeeba is one of those rare people who's been able to affect change in HIV policy in a complex socially conservative context. She's done this by building coalitions across her countries' community, faith, and ethnic fault lines; by bringing divided (and sometimes divisive) groups together to find common ground – the desire to protect Malaysia's young people, for example, or the leadership's desire to provide modern medical care backed by state-of-the-art science. A first and key contribution was work she did with progressive Islamic scholars on exploring a Koranic basis for harm reduction. This proved to be essential as a starting point for reform in Malaysia. It may have relevance for other conservative societies facing similar HIV epidemics. The Middle East and North African region now has the highest rate of new HIV infection of any region globally in 2016 – albeit from a low baseline. So what Malaysia has achieved could have huge impacts on preventing further spread in this tumultuous region. *Insha'Allah.*

Malaysia has also been notable for an increasing openness and willingness to address HIV among other groups at risk, among men and women infected through other modes of spread. The quote above is from the government report on HIV/AIDS in 2015. It acknowledges, correctly, that Malaysia's epidemic has changed. The data show quite clearly that gay men, MSM, surpassed drug users as the group with the largest number of new infections in 2013. The report also addresses transgender women, a group highly stigmatized in Malaysia, the great majority of whom are forced to sell sex, having precious few other choices. And it acknowledges that women selling sex in Malaysia exist, and are at risk. That is progress.

But there are very real reasons for concern. The epidemic overall seems to have peaked in the early 2000s – around 2001. As harm reduction was implemented and people injecting had access to sterile equipment, to methadone, the fall in new infections was initially rapid. The decline flattened in 2010 – and new infections have held steady since. Risks changed. More new infections, about 80 percent, are now from sex, straight and gay, and between transgender women and men. The ministry estimates that 50 percent of sexual transmissions are due to heterosexual sex and 28 percent to sex between men. These percentages represent very different rates in these two groups, however, since gay men account for no more than 2–3 percent of men – so the HIV burden is much greater in this markedly smaller group.

This changing epidemic has proven much tougher to address than prevention and treatment for drug users. Sex work remains illegal in Malaysia. Allegations of trafficking of Rohingya women (and men – mostly for the fishing and seafood packaging industries) from Myanmar into debt-bondage in Malaysia have made the government cautious about policy reforms. And a rising tide of more conservative strains of Islam, seen too in formerly tolerant Indonesia, is raising real concerns about the ability of Malaysia to respond to HIV among MSM. Attempts to force 'effeminate' schoolboys to be more masculine through brutal faith-informed programs are one example. The continued persecution of opposition leader Anwar Ibrahim on sodomy charges is another.

Dr Adeeba is now the first woman dean of a medical school in Malaysia. We are close colleagues and she was, happily, elected to the International AIDS Society governing council during my term as president. Together we co-chaired an IAS consultation on HIV in conservative societies held in Istanbul, Turkey, in February 2016. This fascinating meeting brought together physicians, legal experts, policy makers and community members from across the Islamic world. From Turkey and Malaysia, Iran, Syria, Lebanon, Saudi Arabia, Morocco, Tunisia, Afghanistan, and Central Asia. Prof. Adeeba and I were in a discussion group on Islamic approaches to HIV when we got to the issue of HIV services for gay men. A distinguished Islamic jurist from one of the more conservative states was emphatic that all people living with HIV should be treated with care and respect – no matter how they were infected. I was troubled by this partial answer, since it seemed to imply a religious obligation to care for the sick – but no similar need to provide meaningful prevention for those at risk before infection. During a break, I asked Adeeba if she'd raise the prevention issue, sensing (a good rule with Adeeba in the room) that this would go over much better coming from her than myself. She did a graceful job. The judge was not happy to be pressed. He said Prof. Adeeba was asking him to condone these kinds of relationships. No, that was something he could not accept. His views would mean ongoing failures of prevention – and the kind of ongoing HIV spread that is maintaining Malaysia's epidemic in this fourth decade of HIV.

1996

On World AIDS Day, December 1, 1995, the Malaysian AIDS Council, an umbrella body of 22 AIDS organizations, commemorates those who have died and those still fighting. A memorial service has been organized by Pink Triangle, one of the largest activist groups. The turnout is eclectic. In this ethnically and religiously divided society, the crowd is a rainbow mix of Malays, Chinese, Indians, and expats. There are women covered from crown to toe with only their faces exposed, eating sweets and drinking tea with girls in miniskirts, short spiked hair and pierced noses. A gay couple, both professionals, staff the information booth. One is Malay, the other Chinese. Several gaunt addicts sniffle against a far wall; social activists from Singapore and Indonesia network with diligence; the divine Khartini Salmah, a Malay transgender outreach worker, dishes out plates of food. Khartini also wears a proper ankle-length shift, but she has *big* hair and *serious* nails. There's a dance performance, several dramatic monologues, and an interview for the national radio with Winston Chu, a Malaysian person with AIDS (PWA) who tells his story with heart-wrenching honesty.

Marina Mahathir is among the first to arrive and the last to leave. She is the chairwoman of the AIDS council,[1] a key fundraiser and organizer. She is also the daughter of the country's long-serving prime minister, Dato Dr Muhammad Mahathir, then head of the United Malay National Organization (UMNO), the party that has ruled Malaysia for nearly four decades. Marina is arguably the most prominent woman of her generation in the country, but she is no figurehead here; these are her friends. Her classy, natural presence draws the media and inhibits the authorities, a happy conjunction.

This gathering, in Southeast Asia at least, could only be happening in Kuala Lumpur (KL). The language is KL English, swift, articulate, and spicy with other tongues. Most of the organizations represented here are service groups, but many are also activist in orientation. The language and symbols in the room, and on people's clothes, are instantly recognizable as part of the international AIDS movement: pink triangles, rainbow flags, the quilt display, red ribbons on lapels, 'silence = death' and 'action = life', ACT UP, Fight Back, Fight AIDS. Many of the people at the memorial service are friends. After places like Burma and Cambodia, it is a great joy to be able to speak freely, to feel understood, to be with gay men who have been part of the world I come from. These are people who can visit Thailand with real passports, unlike Burmese friends; people who can communicate via e-mail.

The same evening, there's a series of one-act plays commissioned from young local writers. It is called 'Talking AIDS'. Each of the short pieces deals with an aspect of the epidemic in Malaysia. It's a pleasure to hear theater in English, to see Malaysian responses and hear Malaysian ideas in the context of a theatrical tradition that's immediately accessible. Some of the plays are pointedly explicit. In the first, a young woman who's had casual sex after a drunken evening takes the audience through a miserable morning-after anxiety attack. In another, a young rough talks on the phone with one of his buddies – a whoring buddy, who's just been diagnosed. One of the best, written by a Pink Triangle member, is the monologue of a public health official, a conservative Muslim, remembering one of her first cases of AIDS, a young gay man who taught her something about, of all things, love. It is a surprisingly sophisticated, complex portrayal; I had expected a lampoon. But this is the Kuala Lumpur of the new Malaysians, and they are *with it*.

They are not, however, in power; UMNO is, and UMNO is defined by single-party rule, a policy of 'positive discrimination' to support the Muslim majority against the economic clout of the Chinese, strict media censorship, and little or no tolerance of political opposition. (They are still in power in 2016.) Compare the KL daily newspapers to the *Bangkok Post* or *The Nation* and you know instantly that the Malaysian print media are only a cut above the unspeakable *New Light of Myanmar* or *The China People's Daily*, full of smiling ministers kissing babies, human interest stories on the virtues of tradition, pages of sports, and advertisements for luxury automobiles. All of which serves to make Malaysia a country of paradoxes, contradictions, and jarringly different official and unofficial versions of events.

The country has done well in development terms; its economic growth has been no less rapid than Thailand's, but investments have been much more evenly distributed. While Thailand has joined the extreme economies of Latin America in terms of iniquitous wealth distribution (it is now one of the world's ten worst countries in terms of the gap between haves and have-nots), Malaysia has steadily raised the living standards of the poor through education and targeted development. The result is an impressively prosperous society, and one where economic opportunity has helped to defuse potent ethnic hostilities, as well as the potential rise of militant Islamic movements. Kuala Lumpur is by far the best managed and most habitable capital city in Southeast Asia. Things work: the roads are a pleasure to drive; the city is full of greenery; the shops are crammed. The recently completed National Mosque is both modern and Islamic: sweeping, harmonious, crisp white lines.

This is not to say that the politics of ethnicity and faith have been resolved, or are anywhere close to declining in importance. The population is approaching 20 million people, and is officially 60 percent Malay (all Muslim, by UMNO definition), 25 percent Chinese (Buddhist, Christian, and Confucian), 10 percent Indian (Hindu and Christian), and perhaps 1–2 percent indigenous and tribal minorities (Animist, Christian, and Muslim). Religion and ethnicity in Malaysia are not just about food preferences and dress. There are government bank loans reserved for Malays; parts of Kuala Lumpur are 'reserved' for Malay ownership; university entrance exams have different admission criteria for different ethnic groups; the Malay language is heavily promoted. All ethnic Malays are officially Muslims, ensuring a majority Islamic population, at least on paper. There is freedom of worship for all groups, but the UMNO is in firm control of the government, and its policies are true to its name: Malay nationalist. This is a country where race, identity, and religion count in almost every facet of public life. And there is some evidence to suggest that ethnicity may be playing a key role in the distribution of HIV subtypes in Malaysia as well, as we shall see.

The government, military, police, and a considerable bulk of the civil service are Malay, and thus Muslim-dominated. The Chinese are the economic power in the country – bankers, industrialists, developers – and they also dominate the professions, academic life, and medicine. The Indians are too few to dominate any sector, but are active in the professions, trade, and small businesses. There is also a considerable population of illegal workers and migrants: perhaps 200,000 Indonesians and 50,000 Burmese. These are the menial and day laborers, loggers, agricultural workers, servants, and the underclass. There is a Thai population here as well, not large, and not very visible, unless you look at HIV cases – many are Thai women working in swanky 'health clubs' and 'fitness centers' that double as discreet sex venues. This reality, however, is as covert in

Kuala Lumpur as it is open in Phnom Penh or Bangkok. Malaysia has many faces. The one UMNO would like the world to see does not include prostitution, or heterosexual promiscuity, or homosexuality. Malaysia's policy on drug use is another matter.

A hard line on drug use is very much a part of the country's identity. As you land on Malaysian soil, the pilot of your aircraft calmly announces, 'Welcome to the Islamic Republic of Malaysia. We have a mandatory death sentence for narcotics trafficking.' And they use it. When I met with the head of Malaysia's national drug enforcement agency (a Malay, one should probably specify here), he showed me the numbers of traffickers hanged, annually, over the past decade. The numbers seemed steady throughout the period, between 175 and 250 per year. I pointed out that if capital punishment were meant as a deterrent, it seemed not to be working. Shouldn't the numbers fall over time? 'Profit, you see. It's just so profitable.' Indeed. But one might add that the mules who carry drugs are mostly 'little people' in desperate need of cash. Hanging them might have little effect on the drug trade.

'Yes. We know this. But we feel very strongly about drug use here.'

'Could needle exchange be used in Malaysia to reduce the spread of HIV among addicts?'

'Yes. But *we* cannot do it. That is for NGOs. As a government body we must enforce the rules that support our national beliefs.'

The system is nothing if not thorough. Police have the right to screen anyone they suspect of drug use with a urine test. Urine is screened for all other routine arrests as well. If the test is positive, you get a mandatory blood test. If that confirms drug use, you get 18–24 months' mandatory incarceration in a drug treatment center. The 'treatment' is cold turkey, as in Burma; no drugs are used to medicate for withdrawal. Does it work? The drug program director said that, unfortunately, many of the admissions were repeat offenders; some had been in and out of treatment three or four times. The failure rate is about 65 percent, and half the yearly arrests are re-arrests. (These figures do not include the many Malaysian PWID who cross the border into Thailand, where drug detoxification is free, voluntary, lasts three weeks, and includes a methadone taper to get you through withdrawal. About half the patients treated each year at the Thai government treatment center near the border are Malaysians.)

All persons found to have positive tests for drug use (opiates, marijuana, and amphetamines) are also screened for HIV. HIV-infected persons are segregated in the drug treatment centers, to 'protect' the others from HIV infection. Condoms are not distributed in these centers, although condom use has been discussed recently (after proposals from AIDS activist groups demanding that men in detention be allowed to protect themselves). The HIV rate among arrested drug users is a steady 15 percent, and has been stable for several years. This is much lower than Thailand, and very much lower than Burma, and probably reflects the greater availability of needles and the higher educational level of Malaysians. This is a somewhat different population of users than in other settings: the majority are employed at the time of arrest, and many are working- or middle-class. PWID are found among all ethnic groups, though the majority are young Malay men. And that is part of the anxiety.

Death sentences for traffickers, mandatory screening for drug use, mandatory two-year incarcerations: put this together and you have a society seriously committed to drug control. It has been this commitment that has shaped Malaysia's response to AIDS.

'Seek and ye shall find' is a motto in public health. If you screen all of one group for a disease, and do not systematically screen others, you will find the problem where you have looked for it. This is a fair representation of the HIV situation in Malaysia. The first reported case was detected in 1986. Most of the early cases occurred among recipients of imported blood products (hemophiliacs) who were systematically screened, homosexual men returning from abroad, and among people who inject drugs (PWID). By December 1995, the time of the World AIDS Day celebration in Kuala Lumpur, 14,418 cases of HIV infection had been reported, and 331 cases of AIDS. The majority of these reported cases, 77 percent, were among PWID. But the great majority of HIV tests had been done on PWID.

However, it is widely acknowledged that there is significant under-reporting of both HIV infections and AIDS cases and deaths. Without systematic studies among people at sexual risk – pregnant women, people attending STD clinics, gay men – it was impossible to know. Such studies were problematic in UMNO's Malaysia. This is an Islamic society still, and there is considerable discomfort with the idea of heterosexual spread of HIV.

Just how uncomfortable was made clear to me in an interview with the Director of the Malaysian National AIDS Program, Dr Harrison Aziza. She told me in no uncertain terms that promotion of condom use was not acceptable in Malaysian society, that HIV vaccines were also unacceptable, and that safer-sex education was definitely not on the national agenda. When I asked what might be acceptable, she warmed:

'Malaysia is leading the way with education. We are not promoting "safe sex", but "right sex". "Right sex" is sexuality in the context of monogamous marriage. We are teaching these values, Islamic family values, to our school children. This is societal prevention for HIV and other STDs. We believe that not only will this prevent HIV, it will also prevent all the other social problems associated with pre-marital sex, extra-marital sex, and other unacceptable sexual behaviors. This is our policy, and we are aware that it is not a Western one. But we are a traditional society, and we have the right to choose our approach to these problems. The West has not done so well with its approaches, so why should we copy them?'

It should be mentioned that Dr Aziza has a Master's degree in public health from Johns Hopkins University and lived, for a time, in Baltimore, a city with very high pregnancy rates in the public schools, a chronic and widespread heroin problem, a homicide rate perhaps ten times that of Kuala Lumpur, and a good many more HIV-infected persons than she currently has to deal with. It is easy to be critical of the UMNO approach. It is much harder to admit the awful shortfalls of our own attempts to manage social problems, unsafe sex among the young, and drug use.

'Do you think there's a place for safer-sex education among people already engaged in sex? I mean sex workers and gay men, for example.'

'Yes, of course. But *we* cannot do it. That is what NGOs are for, to deal with these marginalized groups. Our concern is with the future generation. And after all, these groups are very small in our country.'

Fair enough, I thought as I left her. She had several points. But if HIV was already spreading among adults, would Islamic education of schoolchildren not be too late to stem the tide? Education for schoolchildren could take years to bear fruit, assuming it worked at all. What I did not say, since I was a guest in her office and had not been invited to criticize her proposals, was that there was already a significant body of evidence to suggest that sexual risks in Malaysia were much more common than the government was ready to admit. The Ministry of Health collaborated with the World Health Organization in 1992 in a large survey of the health and behavior of Malaysian adults. This study was the first of its kind in the country, and sought to measure potential vulnerability to sexual spread of HIV. A total of 2,270 adults were interviewed regarding their sexual histories. The majority of married adults, 55 percent, reported having had sex before marriage, and 29 percent had between two and ten lifetime sexual partners, which, if you're familiar with these numbers in other cultures and settings, is impressive. How many had had only one sex partner in their lives? Just 38 percent. Of men who reported ever having had sex, 33 percent said they had had 'casual' sex in the past year. In addition, 11 percent of married men reported extra-marital, casual sex in the past year. Not Sodom and Gomorrah, but not Iran either. In fact, these rates of sexual activity are not very different from reports of Thai behavior, which is why they caused a considerable stir in Malaysian medical circles. Malays tend to see the Thais as licentious and permissive Buddhists. By comparison, their own culture is supposed to be much more disciplined and sexually continent. The WHO survey findings suggest that despite the rhetoric, sexual behavior in the general population of both countries is not as different as the bodies politic would prefer. These findings, it must be said, have not been used to guide government HIV-prevention programs in Malaysia. It may also be true that much of the sex reported in the 1992 study did not actually take place in Malaysia.

Malaysians were then the largest single group of visitors to Thailand, at over a million per year, according to TAT, the Tourism Authority of Thailand. There is discreet prostitution in Kuala Lumpur's red light district, but for many Malaysians Thailand's border to the north offers close and much safer venues for sexual services than their home communities. The Thai border provinces of Hat Yai, Yala, and Songkhla have developed a thriving commercial sex industry geared to these Malaysian (and Singaporean) visitors. This includes not only straight sex but also gay prostitution, live sex shows, erotic shops, the usual tacky trappings of commercial sex in Asia. A 1993 study of 503 sex workers in Thailand working near the

Malaysian border found that 97 percent of their clients were non-Thai nationals, the majority being Malaysians and Singaporeans. These border area sex workers reported that Malaysian men were much more likely to request sex without condoms than were Thai men. Thai men have been bombarded with safer-sex messages, Malaysians have not. There could be cultural differences at work here as well, but again, little is known about the attitudes of Malaysian men to condom use.

The isthmus of Kra is a border zone for Malaysia, Thailand, and Burma. All three nations share it, and it was long contested by England and France. Indeed, the Thais ceded four southern provinces on the isthmus to Britain in the nineteenth century, and these now make up Malaysia's four northernmost states. The Burmese port of Mergui on the isthmus was also Thai until the nineteenth century. What has now developed is a new 'triangle trade'. The cross-border sex purchasers are Malaysians, the businesses are owned and run by Thais, and the sex workers are overwhelmingly Burmese women and girls, trafficked from Burma's zones of civil war and poverty. Conditions are appalling. Many of the women are debt-bonded slaves. This may not be what ASEAN has in mind when its foreign ministers talk about 'regional initiatives', but it is a reality, fueled by Malaysia's puritanism, Burma's hungers, and Thailand's expertise in offering tourists what they want but wouldn't dare purchase at home.

This triangle has already produced an AIDS disaster for Thailand and Burma, and is likely to do so for Malaysia as well. On the Burmese side, the isthmus port of Kawthaung reported the highest rates of HIV among men attending STD clinics of any region in Burma: over 30 percent in 1995. The Thai province with the highest rates of HIV in the general population, after those in the far north of the country, is Ranong, at the northern edge of this southern border zone. It would be a miracle if HIV did not cause similar problems in Malaysia, especially given the reluctance of Malay men to wear condoms. Until the Malays begin to screen the general population, however, this will remain unknown.

One piece of this puzzle has recently come to light, through an unexpected set of findings. Because HIV has multiple subtypes, finding different subtypes in different groups in a population can tell us something about how HIV is spreading. The classic example is again

Thailand, where the B subtype of HIV, the predominant virus in the West in both gay men and drug users, accounted for the majority of infections among Thai drug users. In contrast, the explosive spread of HIV among sex workers was largely due to subtype E, suggesting that there was not one epidemic in the country, but two, and that they were not tightly linked, at least initially. Until recently, the HIV subtypes circulating in Malaysia were little studied. On two trips to Kuala Lumpur, however, we were given serum samples from the country's blood banks, STD clinics, sex worker clinics, hospitals, and drug treatment centers – about 90 specimens in all. The Walter Reed group studied these for subtype variation, and a fascinating picture quickly emerged. There were again the same two subtypes as in Thailand, but they seemed to cluster not only by risk group (B was more common among drug users, E among those infected sexually and among sex workers) but also by ethnic group. The Indians (all men) had only B, the Malays had an equal mix of B and E, and the ethnic Chinese and Thais had mostly E. Disturbingly for the Malaysians who would resist such findings, about 40 percent overall were not drug users, and about 10 percent of subjects were infected prostitutes working in KL itself. This is a small study, but it is nonetheless a warning; sexual spread of subtype E in Malaysia looks very much as in Thailand. Drug use is not the only issue for Malaysia, however limited the information on heterosexuals.

A further limitation on understanding HIV/AIDS in Malaysia is the lack of information on the sexual behaviors and risks of men who have sex with men. Despite the efforts of groups like Pink Triangle, sex between consenting adult men is a felony in Malaysia, and heavily stigmatized outside cosmopolitan KL. Like so many former British colonies, Malaysia's laws still specify harsh sentences for the heinous crime of 'buggery', that peculiar anal obsession of the British, who felt the need to criminalize it throughout the world. But we should not (however enjoyable it is to do so) bash Britain too much on this score; some of the Malay states are administered under *Sharia*, Islamic law, in addition to Victorian anal fetishism, and *Sharia* heavily penalizes gays and lesbians. Such laws and penalties make self-reporting of gay or bisexual risks unlikely. Hence nearly all positive cases not ascribed to drug use are listed as either 'heterosexual' or 'unknown' risk categories. It seems contradictory in a country where AIDS activists are so sophisticated, and urban gays so accepted, that gay sex should still be so criminalized. But Malaysia is much larger than KL. And UMNO is unlikely to adopt policies that would risk the ire of the traditional Muslims. In the U.S., President Clinton quickly abandoned his support for gay rights out of political expediency. Malaysian gays are fed to the same lions, to keep them busy, and from turning on their keepers.

This confusion over risks is not limited to gays. All drug users here are assumed to be sexless, to have no HIV risks other than their drug habits. If true, this would make them unique: in most countries addicts have greater sexual risk for HIV than others, given their poverty and chaotic social lives, and the need to sell sex for drugs. But if you test positive for drugs and for HIV, you got HIV through drug use. Period.

Medicine The University of Malaya, in Kuala Lumpur, was founded by the British, and it continues to be an English-language institution. The National University, just down the road in the same comfortable suburb of Petaling Jaya, is a Malay institution, founded after independence in the 1960s. They both have undergraduate- and graduate-level programs, medical schools and teaching hospitals. But it is the University of Malaya that has taken the lead in AIDS: this is where the national HIV lab is, and where a good number of Kuala Lumpur's PWAs come for care. It is a beautiful facility. The campus is large and modern, with spacious lecture halls and quality laboratories. Nearly all of the senior medical faculty are ethnic Chinese. Their academic work is world-class, their English flawless, but guarded. The tension between these academics and the government, on whom their budgets depend, is real. A professor of medicine explained how the system of medical admissions works. It is a reasonable example of the kind of accommodations Malaysians are used to making.

Malays are under-represented in the field of medicine, which is currently dominated by Chinese and Indians. Students take their medical school qualifying exams together, and they are scored identically, but the admission criteria are set later, and these are based on ethnicity. A Chinese student in a given year must score more than 90 percent, for example, while Malays achieving 80 percent will be admitted (the exact criteria vary from year to year, and are kept secret). This is done to ensure that the next generation of physicians will be more Malay, less Chinese. Students who still want to be doctors can go overseas, to Australia or the Philippines, for medical education, but they have to do this privately. The system is called 'positive discrimination' and it is really very similar to the U.S. policy of 'affirmative action', although it is aimed at a majority population, not minority ones. Some of the same negative effects are evident. You cannot help but think that the Malay students are there because of their race, not their ability. It also means the Chinese who do make it are immediately thought to be particularly gifted. Such programs may do much to address imbalances in numbers, but the psychological effects of discrimination, however 'positive', or 'affirmative', are more pernicious.

While the Malaysians may be resistant to investigating some aspects of HIV spread, and while laws against drug use and homosexuality may be harsh, and the medical system discriminatory, there is no question that for a Southeast Asian with HIV infection, Malaysia is a much better place to be than almost anywhere else. The clinics and hospitals are by far the best equipped that I have seen. There is no mistaking the investments that have been made in medical infrastructure, education, and advanced training. The national blood bank is state-of-the-art and superbly run. Malaysia, perhaps alone in the region, has the will and resources to pay for decent HIV/AIDS care. It may need these resources. If sexual spread follows the Thai pattern, or if it is already under way and simply not yet detected, there could be many more cases than the government has planned for. Given the progressive medical community, Malaysia's committed activists, and the capability already present, there are more reasons to be hopeful than not. And Malaysia does at least offer an example of an ethnically complex post-colonial society committed to coexistence and co-operation. It's *holding*.

7 | VIETNAM: HARM REDUCTION IN THE BALANCE

> I was gambling and lost money; I fell into despair, losing confidence. Then my friends said to me that drugs can help stop sadness and despair, life will become happy again. At the beginning, I smoked opium just a little. Then I injected it. Gradually, I began using every day and I don't know when I became addicted to drugs. It lasted for over one year then I quit. However, I can't believe that now I have to pay such a high cost. (A former law student and army veteran, now a cyclo driver in Ho Chi Minh City)

Peace has been good for the people of this beautiful country. Vietnam in 2016 enjoys a hard won, moderate prosperity. With a population of over 90 million souls, she has become a major exporter of food (rice and seafood). Per capita income was estimated at about U.S.$3,500 last year. Life expectancy, probably the most important single measure of well-being, has risen steadily. And the population has gone through the demographic shifts associated with rising prosperity; the leading causes of death in 2010 were cancer, followed by stroke, and then heart disease – the killers of modernity, of aging. HIV was number nine out of ten, accounting for 3 percent of adult deaths, ahead of diabetes, but behind tuberculosis and road injuries (both at about 4 percent).

But peace has not delivered freedom – this is still a single party state, and that party is the authoritarian communist one which seized control after the hard fought victory over the U.S. (and the French before that.) This is a highly centralized state, though one demonstrably capable of enacting reforms.

Vietnam's HIV epidemic is still largely related to needle sharing among the country's large population of people who inject drugs. PEPFAR estimates of the number of people living with HIV at some 250,000 in 2014, the majority of whom were injecting drug users.

And they still account for about 60 percent of all new HIV infections. Drug policy and the party's ability or inability to reform it have been determinative in the shape of the epidemic.

In the 1990s Vietnam was known for some of the most hardline drug policies in Asia. Drug trafficking carried the death penalty, and this included petty traders, usually drug users themselves at the bottom of the trade. Drug treatment, such as it existed, was based on the forced labor model in the country's highly controversial 06 Centers. In 2011 there were 123 of these 06 Centers nationwide, with about 25,000 people held in them on any given day. A recent Brookings report by James Windle described the 06 Centers (and called for their closure):

> The majority of 06 Center inmates are arrested by the police or delivered to the centers by family members. Local authorities can sentence individuals to a maximum of two years' imprisonment in the center, although the incarceration period can be extended by up to two years for post-treatment monitoring and management if the individual is seen as being at risk of relapse.
>
> 06 Centers have been heavily criticized as ineffective and contrary to human rights norms. Inmates are widely reported to be beaten with sticks and electric batons for violating rules or attempting to escape. The homeless are often arrested and sent to 06 Centers to fill police quotas. Since clinical care is poor and treatment is not based on best practices and scientific evidence, relapse rates are high. In fact, 06 Centers strongly resemble labor camps: 'treatment' is centered on 'labor therapy', such as the processing of cashew nuts or sewing cloths, in conjunction with detoxification, performance of military drills, and chanting of anti-drug slogans. Furthermore, post-release support services are limited, and the stigma of being an 06 Center inmate often makes it difficult for users to reintegrate back into their communities, find work, and access health care.

Forced labor, military drills, and chanting slogans are not effective treatments for drug dependency. Neither are they effective HIV prevention. Indeed, the Brookings report goes on to share evidence that the HIV acquisition risks may actually be higher in the 06 Centers than in the communities from which the detained come. This is because while drugs are more scarce inside than out – sterile equipment is even scarcer, as are condoms – making these dangerous places indeed to be held.

The 06 Centers posed a significant dilemma to the PEPFAR program when Vietnam was chosen as the only state in Asia among the initial 15 countries in 2003. (There is a great back story to this choice, shared by a friend who at the time was serving in a senior position in the Bush administration and who was with the president as he made his selection. India and China were both on the final shortlist. The president is reported to have said 'These countries could pay for these programs themselves if they wanted to. I want to spend this money where money is the problem.' Vietnam it was.) It was unclear if the White House was fully aware what it had taken on. This was the only country selected with an epidemic primarily affecting people who injected drugs. PEPFAR would soon find itself supporting a large methadone program as part of its HIV efforts with the socialist republic.

The country began to change from ineffective policies and toward use of methadone and needle and syringe exchanges with the enactment of the 2005 'Law on HIV/AIDS Prevention and Control' which legitimized both policies. But police and law enforcement continue to harass and arrest drug users. Those who've been in detention, including in 06 Centers, are reportedly less willing to use services like needle and syringe exchanges since this can be used against them as evidence of relapse – and that can lead to prison.

Vietnam is no longer a significant producer of either opium or heroin. The government crop eradication program, though brutal, was successful. Laos and Burma remain the main suppliers for the market in Vietnam. On a trip to Laos I saw poppy fields in districts just a few miles from the Vietnamese border – sparsely patrolled in the rugged mountains they share. In 2014, Vietnamese officials intercepted two tons of heroin smuggled from Laos – and sentenced 29 people to death for smuggling it.

Why heroin? Why in Vietnam as prosperity increases and the wounds of war fade?

1996

Heroin, as a colleague of mine in Baltimore – herself a recovering addict – told me, is a drug used to treat otherwise unbearable feelings, like emotional pain, hopelessness, rages that cannot be expressed, failures that cannot be rectified, grief that cannot be faced. The deeper you go into the cycle of relief provided by opiates, the deeper the darkness when you can't get a fix. As the cost of the drug eats away at every aspect of an addict's life, the losses mount, the pain increases, and the dose needed to keep the pain at bay increases in turn. All the opiates, including heroin, mimic natural brain compounds called endorphins. Due to this biologic affinity with the human brain, these compounds develop intensely strong physical, as well as emotional, craving. The daily cycle of pain and release, the habit and the physical craving, eventually enslave the user in dependency. Treatment is difficult. Most addicts fail an average of four to five attempts before they succeed in quitting. Many do not succeed. One of the effects of opium is to reduce the urge to breathe. (This gives an idea of how deep into the nervous system these agents penetrate; the urge to inhale is as old as the first attempt of life to leave the sea.) When the spiral of use reaches the point where the addict needs huge doses to find relief, the urge to breathe can be suppressed altogether; the quiet death of an overdose is the result, an effect for which morphine has long been used in assisted deaths.

Unbearable pain. Rage that can't be expressed. Hopelessness. To have been on any side of the Vietnam conflict has generated these kinds of emotional states in veterans, survivors, refugees, and former prisoners of war. Americans who fought here had higher rates of heroin addiction than the veterans of any other American conflict. (The Nixon administration implemented a humane methadone program for returning troops with drug dependency for these returning troops – one of the first large-scale methadone programs in the U.S.) Some of this was certainly due to availability, since Vietnam had heroin, and it was practically non-existent for U.S. troops in Korea, or in France in the 1940s. But some of this addiction has also to do with pain. Vietnamese veterans are also susceptible. Imagine having fought on the losing side in this war, and then having to stay. The South Vietnamese Army, the ARYN, was huge. By the end of the American war there were more than 400,000 troops, and enormous numbers of men had already died. Some 110,000 officers and

soldiers were arrested after the fall of Saigon, and subjected to re-
education. It was not a bloodbath, as some had predicted: 95,000
or more left the camps alive, to return to a life marked by having
betrayed the nationalist cause. This cannot have been simple. Ho
Chi Minh in the 1990s was a city full of beggars, and not a few of
these were disabled and/or drug-addicted ex-soldiers who were, for
whatever reason, unable to begin new lives in the socialist republic.

You meet many of these men in Ho Chi Minh City (as Saigon
became). I was approached several times a day by Vietnamese men
looking for Colonel Bob or Captain Pete, their old unit commanders.
Here, uniquely in my experience, people wanted to know how old
I was, precisely how old. When I told them, they usually smiled
diffidently and walked away: too young to have been a part of their
war. Many of these men are still waiting for deliverance from the
communists. It was a shock to discover how much they missed their
American contacts, how much like Americans they were, to hear the
accents and phrases of the American south, or midwest, circa 1970:
'Shit yeah, buddy. We'll catch you later.'

But they didn't. For many, heroin was a way to deal with the loss,
or the losses. And now it has led, for one-third of the drug users here,
to HIV, a much more difficult death than the breathless sleep of an
overdose.

Winds of change   Old Saigon was a sexually permissive place, if only
because the massive foreign presence created such a large market for
sexual services. The Vietnamese people, however, have traditionally
seen their culture as sexually conservative, and communism is always
prudish. The actual sexual practices of the general public in Vietnam
have been little studied under the communists. After the long years
of war, Vietnam went into an extended baby boom; family planning
was not given great attention; the population is now over 90 million
and expanding rapidly. Vietnam is already one of the most densely
populated nations in Asia. The government has had to respond, and
initiated a two-child-only policy. The government-issue condoms
(Vietnam manufactures its own) are called 'Happy Family', and their
logo is a family of four: mother, father, one son, one daughter.

But the government is concerned. How much sexual risk is there
in Vietnam? How much prostitute use? How many married men have
sex outside the family? Their anxiety, which is openly discussed, is

that sexual activity in Vietnam may be more like the Thai example than they think, and that a heterosexual epidemic could follow the outbreak among addicts, much as it did in Thailand, and devastate the population. The Health Ministry in the 1990s was determined to prevent this, and actively studied the Thai response. The Thai program's successes were due, in part, to the fact that Thai sexual behavior *had* been studied before the epidemic. Vietnam was just starting this process. The first major survey, done in collaboration with CARE International, confirmed some of these anxieties. Vietnamese men, northern and southern, *do* patronize sex workers, especially before marriage, on a fairly frequent basis: about one-third of all young men interviewed had paid for sex in the last year, and perhaps one-fifth of married men had done so. In another CARE-supported study of urban men, 54 percent of 1,100 interviewed reported sex with two or more partners in the previous two weeks. That is a lot of sex. Sex with other men was also reported fairly commonly; about 7 percent of men reported having had sex with another man; most of these men were married. But what was more disturbing was the lack of communication these men reported with their wives and girlfriends. Almost none had discussed extra-marital sex with their wives. Extensive focus-group discussions with married women, also done by CARE, found a commonly shared sense of powerlessness, an inability to confront husbands about their behavior. Fear of violence, of desertion, and of HIV, was widespread, a situation strikingly like that of women in Thailand, many of whom also live in fear of contracting HIV from their husbands and also feel incapable of discussing these fears with their men.

Whatever else can be said about highly centralized governments, they can mount impressive national campaigns. If Cambodia in the 1990s represented the difficulties of HIV prevention in a chaotic social order, Vietnam was an example of how a pervasive state can reach every corner of a diverse country and get a message out. HIV prevention was one message the Party embraced. Vietnam 1996 was a country studded with AIDS information, at traffic circles, on billboards, in the papers. In Hanoi, I visited the National Offices of the campaign and saw their current output. The fliers and posters have come a long way from the early 'AIDS kills!' message of just a few years ago. One showed a very loving and tender photo of two men in bed, with an admonition for men to use condoms as a way of showing love. Another was an explanation of what HIV looks like in the early phases, with a photo of a late beloved friend, the beautiful Tina Chow, in the asymptomatic stage of HIV. Tina was one of the first Asian-American supermodels, and later a jewelry designer. She is one of the most prominent American women to have been felled by AIDS, and as fitting an image for the pathos and beauty of lost lives as could be imagined. HIV education partly followed the Thai model, going into schools, workplaces, and the mass media. But whether relations with sex workers, with men in gay bars, or with addicts, were as intimate and supportive is another matter. This was not known. Given the party's legalism and puritanism, it was unlikely. Official documents and educational materials still focused on the 'control and eradication of social evils'.

Hanoi   Ho Chi Minh City, and to a lesser extent Hanoi, were already a bit like Bangkok: big and bustling and growing at dizzying speed, too fast, perhaps, for the liking of the party. Like China and Laos, Vietnam's Communist Party is still very much the only political power in the land. To be part of China's highest elite you have to have been on the Long March. To be a part of Vietnam's, you have to have cut your teeth fighting the French or the Americans. This means that the men in question are no longer young. The current balance of power is toward the reformers in the party, but this could change. There is talk of promoting younger men and women to positions of power. But the Eighth Party Congress, in June 1996, opted for continuity rather than change. The politburo simply closed the country to tourists during the Congress, as though their workings still required secrecy in the age of CNN. That this would be a disaster for the thousands of small business people who were reliant on the growing tourist trade was not a consideration. Most of the tourist trade (and small businesses) are in the south. The elderly men calling the shots are not.

The contrast between the conservative leadership and lives on the ground was striking. In Hanoi I never left my hotel without being offered a woman for the night by cyclo drivers, cabbies, waiters, or barmen. I don't know if the locals can afford the sex, but for a Western man it is depressingly easy to find.

In Hanoi I spent some time with a doctor friend who had visited our project in Thailand. Dr B was a young and talented physician, his wife a nurse. Both civil servants. Together they earned about U.S.$70 a month, barely enough to eat. They were helped along by Dr B's mother, a retired teacher of English, who had a small state pension. Dr B, his wife, his mother, the couple's two children, and a nephew they were helping to raise lived in one room in Hanoi. It was the front room of their family's old house. The family was passionate about education. Though his mother was a widow with very limited resources, she saw her son through medical training on her teacher's salary. Dr B could make more with a private clinic, but he was dedicated to research on dengue fever, and this required his staying at his institute, which receives help from Sweden, and was arguably the best hospital for infectious diseases in the country. (The Swedes and the Finns were the only Western nations to support health care in North Vietnam during the war with the U.S.) Dr B remained grateful for their help. He hoped to do advanced training himself, but was already saving for the education of his children and his nephew.

Dr B was a child during the bombing of Hanoi.

'Yes, it was very frightening. We hid in the basement when the bombs came. We had to try to keep going to school. My mother kept trying to go to work. Once I was alone when a heavy raid came to this neighborhood. I will never forget it. Some of my school friends died. But that is all in the past. We are free now and we have better relations with America, which we want. I don't like thinking about pains and fears from the past. They are behind us. Better that way! We have to go forward and develop our country.'

What did Dr B think about the HIV problem in Vietnam?

'We are going to need help. We are weak in epidemiology. My professor here is very good but he studied in Hungary, all of his books are in Hungarian. Difficult! We have to get more software, learn to analyze on computers. We have a long way to go. This HIV problem is very new to us; people are still very limited in their understanding. We know so little about what is happening in the countryside. I know we will see cases in children. We will. But we're not sure we will diagnose these correctly. And we are not sure we can afford to treat them. You have to understand how poor a country is Vietnam.'

Societies in transition are, by definition, unbalanced. They can be both hopeful and threatening. Rapid growth is painful. Injustices resolve, if they do, unevenly. Thailand had made strides in freedom of thought and speech, but its legal system lagged dangerously, and its police were unreformed and corrupt. Vietnam is not hungry, there are more 'things', but the life of the mind and the life of the spirit remained fettered. The Communist Party has the infrastructure, and the people, to mount impressive education and health programs, and it has done so. But the spiritual void that drives men and women to heroin, to buy and sell their precious physical selves, is less addressed. And this void will not be easily filled by education campaigns. Or, to use an adage, not by bread alone. Still, Vietnam was acting on AIDS, using the Thai example as a model.

2016

The good news for Vietnam is that she has officially become a middle-income country. The bad news is that means donor support for programs like PEPFAR and the Global Fund have been declining. From a peak of U.S.\$89 million in both 2008 and 2009, the 2014 PEPFAR funding was U.S.\$49 million. That fell to U.S.\$33 million in 2015. More worrisome was evidence that rather than use its own resources to cover for these losses, the government was moving back toward the rehabilitation through labor model. The 06 Centers never truly went away; now they may fill again with unpaid laborers shelling cashews and sewing clothes.

Whether the Party is ready, gay men are emerging from the shadows in Vietnam. The country now has a vibrant scene in Ho Chih Minh and smaller ones is several other cities. As we've seen across the region – HIV has found its conditions for spread met in these networks. At least for now, the rates are lower than in the Thai or Chinese gay communities.

Others remain vulnerable too. Work is now being done on a previously hidden community in the socialist republic, transgender women. A recent study among some 200 transwomen in Ho Chih Minh City, found 18 percent to be living with HIV infection – tragically high. In what has become a despairingly common finding, the majority had to resort to selling sex for a living. Being trans – transgressing against highly conserved gender norms and expectations – still hugely limits opportunities for transpersons across the region. There have to be more options in life than sex work or the beauty business.

The epidemic is changing for (cis-gender) women as well. The proportion of women among newly infected people in Vietnam increased from roughly a quarter of new infections in 2007 to one in three by 2014. The Vietnam Administration of HIV/AIDS estimated the country was experiencing about 14,000 new infections a year, so this is a substantial number of women. Most of these women had no known risk factor for HIV other than having a husband or regular male partner at risk. The government says that fewer than 40 percent of young women know how to protect themselves from HIV infection. That's a reality Vietnam will have to face to bend the curve of HIV in the country.

8 | YUNNAN: CHINA'S SOUTHEAST ASIA

1996

The Province of Yunnan is the cradle of the T'ai language family. The modern Thais, Laos, the Shans of Burma, the Assamese, and the ethnic Dai who still live in Yunnan are all branches of this T'ai linguistic tree. The region in southern Yunnan called Xishaung Banna by the Chinese, and Sip Song Pan Na by Thai speakers, is held to be the birthplace of the T'ai. 'Sip Song Pan' means twelve thousand, 'Na' means fields, so this is the land of 12,000 (rice) fields. (Lan Na, the old name for northern Thailand, is the 'million rice fields'.) Northern Thais, but not central Thais, can still be understood in this part of Yunnan if they use their old dialect. This linguistic connection, and the cultural and historical links which years of political isolation have not destroyed, are taking on new importance as Yunnan is increasingly drawn into the development plans of the Southeast Asian community.

What unites Yunnan, Tibet, Burma, Laos, Thailand, Cambodia, and Vietnam is the great Mekong River. In Yunnan it is called the Lancang, an echo of the Kingdom of Lan Xang (million elephants), which once controlled much of what is now southern Yunnan and Laos. The Silk Road followed the Mekong through Yunnan, the Shan states, and across Laos to Huay Sai where it delved into Thailand. This route once brought traders from across Asia into Thailand. Chinese laborers now use the Mekong to get to Laos to find work. This old leg of the silk route carried perhaps 40 percent of the world's heroin in 1996, from Burma and Laos into Yunnan. The route links the Burma road with the China road, crossing the Mekong on the Burma–China border near Kachin state. It is along this route that 80 percent of HIV infections in China had been found, and 60 percent of all China's reported AIDS cases. Most of the infections were among young rural men; heroin addicts of the Kachin, Wa, and Dai (T'ai) ethnic minorities. Further south, in Sip Song Pan Na, the HIV cases were in ethnic Dai girls who had returned from sex work in Thailand. The fact that these girls spoke a dialect close to northern Thai, coupled with their poverty and lack of education, made this part of Yunnan a trafficking center for the sex industry. Taken together, these links suggest that the one major HIV outbreak China had seen by 1996 was very much a part of the wider Southeast Asian epidemic. Yunnan, because of its history, location, and its ethnic peoples, was showing its true face to China in the mirror of AIDS; it was not a Han face.

Once a road, a river route, or a border opens, all manner of things begin to flow. In this region, guns, girls, antiques, heroin, rice, labor, jade, timber, rhino horns, tiger parts, tribal people in search of land: the list is a long one. Two years before virtually all the antiques in the markets of Chiang Mai were Shan. Whole Shan temples, dismembered and split into lots, were turning up in dealers' shops. At the same time, nurses in clinics in northern Thailand were reporting that many of the new sex workers turning up with STDs were Shan women and girls, mostly from around Keng Tung. The border was unofficially open, and the road from Keng Tung to Tachilek to Mae Sai on the Thai side was newly passable. The beautiful Shan Buddhas were corning in the same trucks as the women.

In the dry season of 1994, curious wooden Buddhas with elongated ears, arched eyebrows, and serene smiles began to appear. These were folk carvings, not the highly finished Shan bronzes. While the carving work was often delicately done, the proportions of the figures were eccentric: heads too large, the hands and feet clumsy imitations of Thai–Lao classical styles. Some were absolutely lovely, the folk elements adding both charm and spirituality. Where were they from? 'Thai Lue' was the answer from the dealers, from the Dai ethnic villages in Yunnan. Within a month of the appearance of the folk Buddhas, the nurses were again calling to say that a new group of girls and women were appearing in the clinics. Where were they from? Thai Lue, from Yunnan. Another route had opened, and a new trade in treasures, alive and not, was under way.

Not surprisingly, the countries of the Mekong region then called the river and its surrounding countryside a development zone. Plans included linking (with roads) northern Thailand, the Shan states of Burma, western Laos, and Yunnan, into a 'golden quadrangle' development area. The Asian Development Bank was then supporting the idea, and the ASEAN states had done so as well. Perhaps development of this region will mean that legal goods and tourists, rather than heroin and young girls without passports, will travel the roads of the quadrangle. But the linkages may just as well mean that the last tigers, the last Buddhas in their village shrines, the last villages unreached by traffickers, will lose the protection of isolation and join the great regional boom, never to return.

China proper, by which I mean the Han lands and not the colonial holdings of the Party, also has an HIV problem, but the extent of HIV spread in the Middle Kingdom is currently a guessing game. This was all to change soon.

At the 1995 China International Symposium on AIDS, held in Beijing in a bitter December, the numbers flew about like snow flurries, impossible to grasp. The official figure of reported cases was about 1,700, which everyone agreed was a gross underestimate. The WHO estimate was 10,000, based on a very low rate in what is a gigantic population. This figure was the result of work done by Dr James Chin, a respected researcher who was one of the participants. The Chinese Ministry of Health estimate was 100,000 HIV infections in 1995, based on little evidence, educated guesswork, and the bureaucrat's love of a round figure. A thousand? Ten thousand? A hundred thousand? After much discussion, a Party elder weighed in. The official estimate was to be 100,000 cases by 1995. Fact by decree.

When dealing with HIV in a population the size of China's, it may not matter how many cases you think there already might be – what can matter much more is how common the risk behaviors for HIV infection are among young adults. Is there much prostitution? How much injecting drug use is there outside Yunnan? How many gay and bisexual men are there? What is condom use like? How safe are medical procedures, the blood supply? But none of these questions is any more answerable than the estimates. And some, like the extent of prostitution or male–male sex, are questions with enormous political weight in China. If there are answers, who will be allowed to know them?

China has a very long history of sale and trade in women. In addition to outright sex workers there were always grey zones where sex and financial support were linked: minor wives, concubines, servants, the debt-bonded, slaves – all could be seen as part of a profoundly patriarchal system of the use of women for men's pleasure. To their credit, the communists saw this system as feudal and exploitative.

One of their first social programs after consolidating power in 1949 was to 'eradicate' prostitution. Some four million women were 'rehabilitated' after deliverance from feudal orders. There is some evidence that this extreme program came close to eliminating STDs in China. Certainly prostitution, to whatever extent it continued to exist, became relatively rare when compared to the Warlord or Nationalist periods.

All of this was changing in the economic explosion of China in the 1990s. Everyone needed money, wanted money, wanted it now. Women with beauty were selling it again. Hotel lobbies are full of hostesses; bars and nightclubs had leggy women in short dresses working the crowd; Karaoke waitresses were 'available', and Karaokes were everywhere. Traffickers were back and milking the rural poor for their daughters. Cross-border trade in women and girls was a reality. At the symposium, scattered bits of data suggested that syphilis, gonorrhea, herpes, and several other diseases spread through sex were coming back as well. This phenomenon was quite predictable, and likely to increase, despite the resistance of the Party to sexual behavior outside monogamous marriage. The one-child policy had skewed China's population strongly in favor of males; the youngest age groups were then at something like 106 boys to every 100 girls, and thus the demand for women exceeded the supply. Men will be increasingly willing to pay for sex, as the odds on their finding a wife decline. Just as important was the need to appear rich and successful, which means providing hostesses for business dinners, and appearing at banquets with a beautiful girl or two on your arm.

Beijing was the showpiece of the China that had as its chief slogan Deng Xiao-Peng's famous 'It is glorious to be rich'. The scale of the new city, imperviously trampling the old one, is monumental. Virtually every corner sports a new hotel, shopping mall, or glistening bank.

At the symposium I met Dr Rosalyn Fon, an Australian whose family is from Hong Kong. Rosalyn ran AIDS Action in Hong Kong, which works with sex workers. She is a medical doctor with training in sexology, and had come to Beijing to find out the scope of the burgeoning commercial sex scene in the People's Republic. If you dreamed of a Chinese lady sexologist, you could not come up with Dr Fon. She is tall (5 feet 11 inches), curvaceous, with a highly set bust framed by Garbo shoulders and long white arms. Complete the vision with a serious pair of legs in black leather, stiletto pumps, a poly fur bomber, a shock of rag-doll red hair, dripping earrings and fire-engine lips and you have Rosalyn. The old PRC cadres literally gasped when she first appeared in a skin-tight mini-skirt at the opening ceremony in the Great Hall of the People.

After the first day's session, we agreed to go out on the town. The *Spartacus Gay Guide* had one listing for Beijing: a disco in the basement of yet another vast hotel. I did my best to dress for the occasion, and strode out of the awful 21st Century Hotel with the glamorous Dr Fon on my arm.

We arrived just before nine, and the place hadn't even opened. The disco shared the basement with a huge bowling alley. Dressed for night-clubbing, we watched bowling, a hypnotically dull game, and talked about Hong Kong. Would she stay after 1997?

'Well, I have an Australian passport, so I can get out if it looks bad. But I'm curious, you know, to see what it'll be like. Most Hong Kong people with money are investing in mainland China. They're really more concerned with their business ventures than with things like a free press and the vote. People are looking forward to not paying taxes to the Brits, I can tell you that. But there is one big worry with the PRC in charge, and that's corruption. Hong Kong isn't perfect, but you really do have to be very clever to get ahead, and the best people *do* get ahead. In China it's still who you know, whose kid you are, and who you can pay off to get promoted. Hong Kong people are worried not so much about communism, which is pretty much dead anyway, but about having some party chief's idiot son in charge of their business.'

On to the Disco. Most of the crowd looked like other Westerners who had read *Spartacus*. There was one rather stunning male couple rocking out on the dance floor. They turned out to be well-heeled tourists from New Delhi (and very much in love). Rosalyn and I met one gay Chinese, actually from Beijing but living in Sydney. I mentioned the rather obvious number of attractive young women in revealing dresses scattered throughout the club.

'Yeah, they're working girls. If a club in Beijing doesn't have them, no customers will come. You find them everywhere.'

'Are they hostesses, or do they sell sex as well?'

'You want one, isn't that lady your wife?'

'No, she's not my wife, just a friend. I'm gay, actually. I'm just interested.'

'Of course, they will go home with you. If they didn't, this place couldn't make any money. Beijing people are very cheap; they don't spend money on drinks like the Aussies.'

Rosalyn listened to all this with a slight, bored smile. She had spent several years trying to get the Hong Kong authorities to acknowledge the scale of sex services in Hong Kong and on the mainland, and this was old territory for her. In the cab going back, I asked her about the commercial sex scene. How extensive did she think it was?

'In China now, all the old status symbols are coming back. It's in the genes! The people here have been denied so much for so long. Now they want it all: cars, luxuries, clothes. Sex is just a part of the money-and-power game. And let's face it, things have never been that great for women in China, even at the height of the communist reforms. HIV is a time-bomb here. Talk to the women in the bars, the young executives, they'll all tell you that you get AIDS only from sleeping with foreigners.'

'What about Hong Kong?'

'Officially there are only a small number of cases. The government likes to think that prostitution is uncommon. I've interviewed so many sex workers, and so many of them have repeated bouts of STDs, it just doesn't jibe with the official reports. Hong Kong does have something of a gay scene, though. There are some clubs and discos. We'll just have to see how things are handled when the transfer happens.'

At the Symposium we met several people who were formidably bright and doing important work in virology, epidemiology, and vaccine research. One was clearly a genius. Dr Yiming Shao had been recommended by a Chinese-American colleague at Johns Hopkins as the key person to meet in Beijing. He was one of the first members of the WHO's technical advisory group on HIV vaccines, and has since developed a collaboration with a German group to develop HIV vaccines in China. After a quick lunch on the second day of the meeting with Yiming, I felt, for the first time in ages, renewed optimism for the vaccine effort. The clarity of his ideas was wonderfully refreshing. He was convinced that a vaccine including core and envelope gene products could protect against HIV. He detailed his study plan; it was cohesive and logical, but also visionary. In the new China, he has official sanction for his work.

My translator at the seminar spoke on the second day. He was Dr Zunyou Wu, a young medical doctor with a Ph.D. from UCLA, and a key member of the team investigating the epidemic of HIV among the Kachin (*Jingpo* in Mandarin) and Wa of Yunnan. He had some extraordinary slides of Kachin heroin users injecting each other with pens, bamboo splits, and razor blades. He later showed me a map of the epidemic in Yunnan. The cases were clustered in just three small districts, all along the China–Burma border. Sixty percent of all the infections in this immense country were in this one tiny area. He also had some slides of the Wa communities. If anything, these people were living in an even earlier epoch than the Wa in Burma, who had been penetrated by Burmese communists in the 1960s. The Wa in Yunnan were still in loincloths, still hunting and fishing in their remote mountains, terribly vulnerable, as tribal peoples often are, to exploitation and drugs. Among the Kachins in Ruili, the border district in Yunnan, 17 percent of young men on either side are drug users, according to Dr Zunyou.

Information on the mandatory 're-education' programs used by the Yunnanese authorities to treat ethnic addicts was not available. It seemed however, not to be working. Certainly the HIV data shows an epidemic in poor control, and there are already a number of pregnant women – wives of addicts – infected. Still, it was nowhere near as grave a situation as in Kachin state on the Burmese side, where 91 percent of addicts tested HIV-positive in 1995, and where the virus had already leapt out of the addict circle and into the general population. This was not what the beleaguered Kachins needed as they struggled with the junta to the south, and China to the north.

Would what was happening among the ethnic minorities in Yunnan going to affect the Middle Kingdom? China was still not a very mobile society: people wait years for apartments; lovers postpone marriage for years until they can manage to get jobs in the same city. Social and sexual mixing of the Han and the ethnic populations was still uncommon. Tribal Wa, only a generation away from their last headhunts, were probably not going to work as Karaoke hostesses in Shanghai, at least not in any significant numbers. The greater threat to China was its own resurgent sex industry, its new consumer society, and its rapidly widening disparities in income, which will make selling sex attractive to the poor. With China's strict family-planning laws and extensive network of contraceptive services, it was somewhat ahead of the game. But the future was not at all certain.

2016

Snakeheads and a heroine   The thick manila envelope arrived in my office mailbox in early 1999 with an unusual looking postmark. From Beijing, China, but addressed to me in English in an unfamiliar hand. In it were Xeroxed copies of several documents, some of which looked like U.S. diplomatic cables, others like trip reports. They contained details of HIV, hepatitis, and syphilis infection rates among men and women in Henan Province, China. There was also a fairly detailed investigative report, clearly by someone trained in public health, that again contained very worrisome data from Henan Province, but also from five other provinces, all in central China's Han heartland. This document detailed the risk factors for HIV infection among rural adults in Henan. They were virtually all blood donors. Not recipients of blood products, like hemophiliacs, who had suffered terrible burdens of HIV infection before we had developed tests for the virus and cleaned up blood supplies. But donors. Donors are usually the lowest risk people in a population. Most strikingly, the report had several tables where people were put into groups based on the number of times they'd donated. As their history of donating (or selling) blood increased, so did their likelihood of having blood-borne infections, HIV, but also hepatitis and syphilis. I had never seen data like these. They went in precisely the wrong direction – normally as you identify people with HIV or hepatitis, they come out of the donor pool, so the rates in repeat donors are lower than first time donors. This looked as though donation itself had become a risk for infection. The numbers of affected looked to be in the several thousands. But the report also made clear that the scale and scope of this outbreak was unknown and might involve many more people.

The blood collection industry was fast growing in China, and was known to be active in the five provinces listed. I looked up what I could on Henan Province. Vast, largely rural, ethnically Han. A place that had been horribly affected by the great famine unleashed by Mao's disastrous Great Leap Forward policy.

There was no note or letter accompanying these documents. After I read through them several times, I sat in my office and played through some probable scenarios. Someone in the U.S. diplomatic or public health corps (I thought perhaps the author of the report on the donors) had put this information together and passed it on to me. Call it a leak, or a whistle blow. It seemed likely too that whoever had sent it felt constrained, doubtless by the sensitivity of the material, from publishing the data or sending it to the media.

Why me? And what should I do with the documents, the data they contained?

The why me question was much more straightforward than the question of what to do next. Our projects on HIV in Chiang Mai had lacked a strong virologic component. To address this gap we asked a gifted Chinese–American virologist at Hopkins, Dr Xiao-Fang Yu, to join our research team. He came out to Chiang Mai in 1995 and we quickly discovered a mutual interest in HIV molecular epidemiology (yes, nerd heaven) but also in Thai food, which Xiao-Fang devoured with sometimes frightening speed and gusto. We subsequently published a number of papers together and did work on the Thai virus that would later inform HIV vaccine work in the region, including Xiao-Fang's own work on vaccine development.

When I came back to Hopkins in 1997, Xiao-Fang asked me if I'd be interested in collaborating on some new research he was doing in Guangxi Province, on China's southernmost border with Vietnam. There was an outbreak of HIV among injecting drug users in the border towns of Guangxi, Pingxiang and Baise, in an ethnic minority area known as the Zhaung People's Autonomous Region. When I learned that the Zhaung were a Diac people, close linguistic and cultural cousins of the Thai, Shans, and Lao, it was an easy yes. We got an NIH grant for the project and subsequently published a number of scientific papers, on this emerging epidemic. The situation in Guangxi was fascinating and potentially important for understanding HIV spread. One viral subtype, the A/E virus of HIV, was coming north from Vietnam into Guangxi, seemingly spread by both needle sharing among drug users and through sex. The entry point was one of China's nine gates – the Vietnam–China border crossing at Pingxiang, a booming border town run as a special economic zone. Pingxiang was literally lined with brothels, all the women working in them from Vietnam, for the truckers who carried goods going north (mostly produce) and south (mostly electronics and manufactured goods). To the west, Guangxi bordered Yunnan

Province, and from there, strains from Burma, B/C variants of HIV, also largely spread among drug users, were heading west into Guangxi. Understanding which viruses might prevail, and why, was a critical question. And of course, trying to prevent further spread was even more crucial. My part of the work was designing the epidemiologic studies and implementing the basics of prevention. It was standing room only when we did a training on safe injection practices for about 50 young drug users – men who would become our peer educators. We had to do the bulk of the training in the morning. After lunch, many of the guys went off to shoot up, and came back loopy and nodding off. This was cutting-edge work at the time. We developed a reputation as a group with strong relationships both with the community and with the government – no small trick in the China of the late 1990s. So this was the why me answer, or so it seemed. And because this work was U.S. federally funded, anyone with access to the U.S. federal funding data (it's public but not so easy to find) would find me quickly and learn about our work on HIV in China. (When conservatives in the U.S. Congress put together their 'enemies list' of immoral U.S. research and researchers in the heyday of the Bush administration, they too found this study. I had three on the list.)

Now what to do? Carl Taylor, a wise man of public health who'd founded the Department of International Health at Hopkins, was alive then, and a personal mentor. He also knew China well, having served as head of UNICEF's mission in China before the Open Door policy of the 1980s. I went to him to discuss the documents. His advice was to seek corroborative evidence – he felt the stack of documents was not enough to go on for a concern of this magnitude. I also went to the head of the Hopkins Hospital blood bank, for more of a read on the actual blood collection data. He found the reports disturbing and affirmed that if true, they suggested an iatrogenic (man-made) epidemic of HIV among blood donors of great severity.

But I was stuck. Where could I get more evidence? And what might happen to my collaborators in Guangxi if it turned out their American research colleague was leaking documents about an iatrogenic epidemic in China's heartland? They would be interrogated at the very least. So I sat on the information for several weeks.

And then, one Sunday afternoon about a month later, the phone rang at home.

'Hello, is this Chris Beyrer? The HIV researcher working in China? This is Elizabeth Rosenthal, sorry for the cold call. I'm the bureau chief for the *New York Times* in Beijing. Do you happen to know anything about HIV cases among blood donors in China?'

This was one of those moments when your gut tells you what to do, and you really have to listen. Libby Rosenthal shared that she was a physician, though now working as a journalist. Based in Beijing with her family, but calling me from a family apartment in New York, since this was a hugely sensitive issue in China and she knew she had to be careful about using any kind of communication from Beijing itself.

I asked her for confidentiality, primarily out of concern for my colleagues in China. If she could assure me that she'd protect me as a source, I'd share everything I knew. Her subsequent investigation into the blood donor epidemic in China was great, ground-breaking journalism. It would break as front page news in the *Times* in 2000, and in a series of powerful investigative stories to follow through 2002. The story is a terrible one.

It began with an astute, retired obstetrician named Gao Yijhe. In the late 1980s, Dr Gao began to see some of her former patients, women who's babies she'd delivered, with strange new symptoms. They complained of weight loss, fevers, sweating at night, diarrhea, skin rashes. Many had husbands who were sick as well, or who had died of similar illnesses. Dr Gao began to suspect that her former patients, improbably, had the new disease she'd heard about, but which was affecting gay men in the West – AIDS. She visited many of the villages and towns from which these women came, and found large numbers of people in these communities sick and dying of the same illness, often in the same family or household. By doing careful clinical work, asking questions, taking medical histories, she was the first person in China to put together the cause of the epidemic, HIV, and the route of exposure: the 'snakeheads'. Henan is poor. Her patients were mostly country people, farmers in crowded impoverished counties. What they shared was that many had supplemented their incomes by selling blood to the snakeheads, blood collectors who paid poor people in fast cash. Dr Gao found 'blood houses', newer and nicer than the old peasant homes, that families had built with the money they'd made. Now many lay sick and dying in those new homes. This was because, as Libby Rosenthal's investigations would later uncover, the snakeheads reused collection equipment to cut costs. To allow for donors to donate more often they reinfused the red cell fraction of the blood, often in pooled fashion. To maximize profits, they had exposed thousands, perhaps many more, to HIV, viral hepatitis, syphilis. And this is why the data I'd been leaked showed so clearly that the risk of infection went up with each donation.

Libby Rosenthal and I eventually nominated Dr Gao for the Jonathan Mann Prize in Health and Human Rights, which she won, to her great joy. But the government of the People's Republic took a very different approach. She was harassed, both of her physician children lost their jobs, and eventually she was forced to seek political asylum in the U.S., where she now lives. Wan Yan Han, the HIV and human rights activist who first put the data on blood donors in Henan on his organization's website, was 'disappeared', for some months, tortured, and released under international pressure, and he too, along with his family, are now in exile in the U.S. These brave people were persecuted relentlessly for their efforts on behalf of the donors and their families. But the men who ran the snakehead system, including the then governor of Henan, went untouched and untroubled. The governor went on to join the politburo, and was, hence, an untouchable in China's system. It was not until the disastrous bungling of the early response to the SARS outbreak that Chinese officials would suffer repercussions for their mismanagement. By then, tens of thousands of rural young people had already died of AIDS.

The current wave   China's AIDS road did not end in Yunnan, or in the border towns of Guangxi, or among the rural poor of Henan, selling their blood at such extravagant cost. It continues, but now in the wealthiest and most developed region of the country, China's eastern seaboard, in Shanghai, Guangdong, Beijing. And like so many of the current epidemics in the region, this one too is exploding among China's young gay men. For the AIDS conference in Washington D.C., in 2012, I led an international team in a massive effort to pull together all the available current data on HIV among men who have sex with men worldwide. We published this in a special themed issue of *The Lancet*, for the conference. The three countries reporting the highest rates of new infection were one we suspected would be there, Thailand, and two that were a surprise; Kenya and China. In

China the baseline was lower than in Thailand, about 3–8 percent of gay men, depending on the city sampled, but the rates of new infection were higher – explosively so in several cities. Since China has the largest gay population of any country on earth (due to her enormous size), this was already a major epidemic in 2012. And it has continued.

Once again, there is a Southeast Asia connection to this latest war in the blood. Thailand was the first country to truly open to tourism from China – it extended visa on arrival to Chinese travelers, and quickly became the most common overseas tourist destination for Chinese. Most were not gay men, of course, but some were. And like their brothers in the conservative and closeted societies of Malaysia, Hong Kong, Taiwan, and Singapore, these men found Thailand affordable, tolerant of same-sex liaisons, and offering a large variety of options for finding sex with men – from saunas and massage parlors to go-go bars and cruising zones. Molecular epidemiology was again helpful in understanding what was happening at viral and network levels – the strains that had been circulating in gay men in the region, mostly the old subtype B that also caused the U.S. and European gay man's epidemics, was being rapidly replaced by the variant found in most Thai gay men, the A/E virus that we have met before. There is actually a silver lining to this otherwise threatening cloud. The one HIV vaccine candidate that has shown any efficacy, in the Thai–U.S. RV144 trial, was developed against this A/E variant. So the next generation of vaccines based on this product can likely be tested in China now, among gay men.

My longtime friend and colleague Yiming Shao, who I described in the first edition of this book, has continued to play leading roles in China's HIV efforts. He invited me to give a keynote on HIV prevention for gay men at China's national HIV meeting, in Shanghai, in November 2015. Yiming's main agenda in this invitation was to have me meet with the leadership and as he said, 'avoid the mistakes the U.S. made in not responding to HIV in the gay community in time'.

I had never been to Shanghai before this, having mostly worked in China's far south, and having made many trips to Beijing to meet the health leadership. Shanghai is famously China's richest city, the cradle of the Open Door Policy and the center of banking, finance, fashion – and gay life. My talk seemed to go well. My translator was a man I'd met on my first trip to China, a distinguished, now retired, professor with a gorgeous command of English. But the meetings with the leadership were a disappointment. I was asked over a very modest banquet lunch (this was the height of Xi Jinping's anti-corruption drive – gone were the extravagant drunken repasts of his predecessors) to lay out what I thought China needed to do to address this new wave of spread. I laid out three steps, following the rule that people rarely hear more than two or three key points. First, expand HIV testing in safety, dignity, and confidentiality, since HIV status awareness is the key to both earlier treatment and to enhanced prevention. This had to be done with the gay community, not to them, as had happened with mass roundups and forced testing in the past. Second, offer immediate treatment to anyone testing positive for HIV infection – and as quickly as possible, since early treatment is better for the individual, and it has a major prevention benefit. Third, for uninfected men at risk, offer PrEP, pre-exposure prophylaxis. All three steps had been taken in San Francisco, and in 2015, this was one of the few places where we could say with confidence that rates of new infection were finally falling in gay men at a population level. The officials listened, polite, attentive, but very quiet. Finally the senior-most man spoke. 'Professor, why won't these homosexuals just use condoms?' That seemed all that was on offer. And we already knew that wouldn't be anywhere near enough.

PART TWO

PEOPLE, RISKS

9 | WOMEN: WIVES, MOTHERS, DAUGHTERS

The basic strategy for the prevention of sexual transmission of HIV for the first decades of HIV comprised three messages: reduce the number of your sex partners (toward monogamy, if possible); use condoms every time you have penetrative intercourse; promptly treat all sexually transmitted diseases (STDs) and reduce (with condoms and partner reduction) your risk of acquiring new STDs. This strategy grew out of prevention efforts by and for gay men, with the 'sex negative' input of bodies like the U.S. Centers for Disease Control (CDC), which were mandated to include promotion of monogamy in its messages. And it worked, albeit with widely varying degrees of success. This triple approach has also had some utility for sexually active heterosexual adults and adolescents, largely in the West, and for sex workers and their clients in many countries. For people with multiple sex partners by choice, HIV risks can be sharply reduced by adhering to consistent condom use and STD treatment.

We have now added to this very limited early toolkit. With the coming of antiretroviral drugs and the expansion of access to treatment, we are in a new prevention era. A landmark multi-country study, HPTN 052, enrolled heterosexual (and a few same-sex couples) where one partner was living with the virus, the other not. In a surprise finding, in about half the couples the woman was the infected partner, not the man. Couples were then randomized to earlier or later treatment – and infection rates in the uninfected partners compared. The results were a rare home run in research – earlier treatment reduced transmission by more than 96 percent. So earlier treatment as a prevention tool for partners is the first addition to the toolkit. A number of other newer tools are in development, including products women might use vaginally, like gels and rings impregnated with antivirals. But only one is ready for deployment for women at risk, oral PrEP. PrEP, pre-exposure prophylaxis with daily oral antiviral drugs (Tenofovir and Emtricitabine, or Truvada) has been shown in several studies to reduce women's risk from HIV-infected male partners. Trials in women at sexual risk more broadly have less consistently shown efficacy, and been made complex to assess due to significant non-adherence to the study medications. PrEP has very real challenges for wide use in women. It requires regular HIV testing since the drugs shouldn't be used if a person does become infected. For PrEP to be meaningful for women, getting tested with partners or husbands, getting counseling as couples, is likely to be essential. For single women at risk, the issues may differ – and carry some of the same stigmas that inhibit unmarried women's willingness to buy or carry condoms. To be seen or known as a woman who needs PrEP. Or to be thought to be HIV-infected, since the medications are the same as many used for treatment.

Imagine yourself a young married woman, in Thailand or Cambodia, Vietnam or Malaysia. You have only one sex partner, your husband. He is your sexual life. Your risks are his risks. You may or may not know what they are. You may or may not be able to ask. 'Reducing the number of sex partners' means not having sex with him, and thus, not at all. This is not an option for many women, no matter what their husband's behavior entails. It would mean giving up having children, an option very few women can accept, particularly among the rural poor, still the majority of Asians, for whom the focus of life itself is the family. 'Use condoms for penetrative sex.' Why? Why introduce condoms into your marriage? Condoms again represent your husband's risks, and again imply reduced fertility. Using them acknowledges that he *has* risks, has other partners, goes to brothels or has a mistress or sleeps with men or injects drugs. And *he* has to put the condom on, has to accept the need to protect you from his behavior. (Thai men, for example, usually report using condoms with sex workers to protect themselves, recognizing their own risk. The acknowledgment that as a user of commercial sex services they could spread HIV to others is unusual.) 'Reduce the risk of STDs' is another ambiguous message for most women. If they get gonorrhea or syphilis, it is, again, their husband's behavior that is at issue. What can a woman do about reducing her partner's risks for STDs, or his need for treatment? This is also true of getting an HIV test, and of being willing to either start antivirals or go on PrEP. To speak of these issues is to suggest infidelity. This can be frightening. It can be deadly.

If these scenarios seems unlikely or uncommon ones, it may be because we're used to thinking of HIV in terms of 'high-risk sex'. Anal intercourse aside, there is no higher-risk sexual activity for HIV than trying to conceive a child. It requires regular unprotected intercourse, the exchange of just those fluids that carry and transmit HIV. Death and life in one ejaculate, a parasitic mechanism of 'fearful symmetry'. Wives outnumber sex workers by many orders of magnitude in all of the countries in this study. Probably in every society. By far the most common risk factor for HIV among women in Thailand is marriage, having one male partner. This has long been true in India, in Burma, and in much of Africa. How else can we explain the report of the Myanmar National AIDS Program that 175,000 pregnant women in Burma were HIV-infected by 1995? These are not addicts, or 'loose women', or sex workers, though a small minority may be. These are women whose HIV exposure comes from just the behaviors their society most strongly supports: marriage, conception, giving birth to children.

We have very little to offer women in these situations. The male condom is problematic. It is strongly associated with prostitutes, 'risky' sex and 'risky' partners, mistrust, and sex without love or commitment. A married woman in Malaysia or Thailand would probably be mortified to buy one. The female condom may be an improvement, but it is expensive, still requires male consent for use, shows outside the vulva, and requires that a woman be willing to insert it. Many Asian women are psychologically unable to touch themselves internally. Many have never had a gynecological examination. *Our Bodies, Ourselves* has not been translated into Shan, or Lao, or Punjabi.

Looking at another gynecological disease may help to illustrate these challenges. Cervical cancer in women is a growing problem worldwide. We now know it is caused by another sexually transmitted agent, HPV, the human papilloma virus, which can cause genital warts in men and women. Women with only one lifetime sex partner are exposed to HPV by that partner. But HPV is tricky, like HIV. HPV-infected men often have no symptoms, although when they do, the warty lesions of penile HPV are unmistakable. In Thai they are called 'Nok Kai', the cock's comb, which they do somewhat resemble, and are one of the few STDs with such a precise folk translation. Cervical cancer is unusual among gynecologic cancers in that we have a cheap and effective screening test, the Pap smear, for early detection. Caught in the first stages, this is a curable disease. Despite the relative ease and low cost of Pap smears, they are rarely done in developing countries. There is now a highly effective vaccine for girls and boys against HPV, but it is expensive, and rarely used in the global South. Most cervical cancer in Thailand, the only Southeast Asian country for which we have reasonable data, is found in later, less treatable stages, or at incurable ones. Pap smears are not done routinely because pelvic examinations are not done routinely. Sex workers get pelvic examinations to look for STDs. Housewives and mothers do not. It should not come as a surprise to find that cervical cancer is the leading cause of cancer death among Thai women – all women, not just sex workers. Or that the HPV vaccine has done little to alter these sad truths.

When we think of protecting women from HIV, now an incurable infection, this reality has to be kept in mind. Limitations on women's health care in much of Asia have already led to a serious failure of prevention for a common and potentially curable disease. HIV will be no easier to prevent than cervical cancer. And, while both diseases are sufficient to kill a woman, their interaction is even more deadly. HIV-infected women progress to cervical cancer more quickly than women without HIV, and HIV-positive women are more likely to infect their sex partners with HPV, since the wart virus can grow without the hindrances of a healthy immune system. The viruses accelerate each other, a phenomenon Dr Judy Wasserheit of the University of Washington called 'epidemiologic synergy'. (This synergy has also led to an increase in the number of cases of a previously rare disease, carcinoma of the anus, among men infected with both HIV and anal HPV.)

HIV exposes women's vulnerability to male sexual behavior. What can women do about it? How will women in Southeast Asia respond?

1996

About 60 women meet each week at a Buddhist temple in Doi Saket district, Chiang Mai Province. Doi Saket was once a rural area, with a small country town and a number of farming villages. Urban sprawl has brought Doi Saket's farmers into the growing suburban economy; land has been sold for sub-divisions; many villagers commute to work in the city; young people leave Doi Saket early, for schooling and for work. These changes have brought some prosperity, but not without costs. The cash economy, and men and women leaving villages for work, have loosened social structures, separated families, changed women's lives. This period of social change, unfortunately, made Doi Saket, and other communities like it, fertile ground for HIV. All of the women who meet at the temple are AIDS widows, many are themselves infected; most are now single mothers. Despite the fact that nearly all of the women in the widows' group were farmers' wives infected by their husbands, community prejudice and discrimination against them and their children has been intense. It was this social ostracism that first brought the group together. They approached the government, who helped them to get support from an Australian donor agency. With the money, the widows of Doi Saket have set up a co-operative, making handicrafts to support themselves and their children. The abbot of the district's central *wat*, who has taken a lead in supporting people with HIV infection, offered the temple grounds for their projects. This is not an HIV prevention program, it is perhaps too late for early interventions here, but it is a way for women to survive the loss of their husbands, to deal with discrimination, and to build solidarity with each other.

The women of a similar community, also in the suburban ring of Chiang Mai, San Sai District, have used another approach. So many young men were dying in San Sai that the community opted for a moratorium on marriage until it was clear which young men would survive the disastrous HIV epidemic in the district. This is probably not going to work, but it represents an incredible change in the social structure of San Sai's villages. Local women know what may happen when they marry – HIV infection – and are opting, at least for the short term, for not marrying rather than risk exposure.

Women's attitudes toward prospective partners are changing as well. In a study among female factory workers in northern Thailand, young women reported that they strongly favored men who did not visit sex workers, and that the sexual history of their potential partners was an important criterion for marriage. This is a sharp change from the attitudes of their mothers' generation, for whom visits to sex workers were often preferred over husbands having mistresses. These were women whose fathers and older brothers traditionally took their adolescent boys to brothels to begin their sexual lives.

The most far-reaching change is a paradoxical one. Young Thai women are increasingly having sex before marriage. The formal term for this emerging pattern is 'serial monogamy'. In serial monogamy, people tend to have only one partner at a time, a steady monogamous partner. But the first, or second, or third partner might not be the one chosen for marriage. Serial monogamy is trial and error, learning, while engaged in sexual relationships, what one wants and is prepared to give to a marriage. This requires contraception, and an awareness on the part of both partners that neither is likely to be a virgin at marriage. It requires empowerment of young women and a seachange for men, who must go from a 'virgin or whore' conception of female sexuality to a partnership with an 'equally experienced and adult' woman.

A striking finding among Thai soldiers was that while condom use was increasing sharply in the early 1990s, and the use of prostitutes steadily declining, the age at first intercourse among these men fell through the same period (from about 16.5 years to 16.1), and the number of men who reported having girlfriends with whom they were sexually active rose. The number of men who reported having had a girlfriend (and not a sex worker) as their first sex partner more than doubled between 1991 and 1995. In other words, young Thai men were still having sex, but they were losing their virginity and having sexual relationships with female peers, not sex workers. Does this mean that these 'AIDS era' young men may establish sexually satisfying lives with their wives? That prostitution will decline due to a fall in demand?

Many Islamic societies believe that sexual desire is a female problem. Women's genitals must be mutilated to prevent them from developing insatiable and uncontrollable craving. Men are seen as much less physical, more spiritual; if men were not constantly aroused by licentious women they would spend their waking hours contemplating the divine. *The Perfumed Garden*, the classical Arabic erotic text, is a paean to women's 'itchy vulvas', their libidinous urges, and the great lengths to which men must go in order to restrain their women. Other cultures have seen this very differently. In Thai culture wives traditionally do not enjoy or initiate sex, and do not have orgasms. Sex workers are for sexual pleasure, wives for producing heirs. A Western colleague and social researcher has done some fascinating work on young women working in factories (women make up about 70 percent of Thailand's factory workers). But it was with her Thai research colleagues that she became intimate enough to encounter the sexual conservatism of middle- and upper-class married Thai women of a certain age. She had her research group to her house for tea near the completion of their project. The subject of sex within their marriages came up. Every one of these women was shocked when my friend mentioned that she and her husband had a satisfying sexual relationship. What did she mean? That her husband was satisfied? No, she explained, she meant that she was satisfied; her husband was a generous partner. She had orgasms. *Orgasms?!* Impossible. Women couldn't have orgasms. How could they ejaculate? The Westerner insisted that women did have orgasms, and there was considerable scientific evidence to prove it. (The Thais present were all educators, physicians, or pharmacists.) When she maintained that she enjoyed sex, the consensus was that there was something very wrong with her. One colleague suggested therapy, while another thought she should take up meditation, to calm her over-aroused senses.

But the daughters of these women might tell you a very different story, one that has been profoundly affected by AIDS. Sexual equality (serial monogamy for both partners until a good match is found) may seem an unlikely outcome of the HIV epidemic in Thailand, but it is increasingly being practiced by young women who want to be a part of their husbands' erotic lives, not just dutiful and sexless mothers of children, who want to know their husbands' and their own risks, and want protection. And their husbands come from a new generation of young men, who have had their sexual debut with a girlfriend, not in a brothel.

This may sound like a change for the better. And perhaps it will be, in the long term, a partial solution to the related problems of the sex trade and sexually unfulfilling marriages. But it was having another consequence in the Thailand of the 1990s. The large pool of young men infected with HIV during the Thai boom (a similar situation prevailed in Burma and Cambodia, where the booms continue) was now marrying. Young women in these countries were selecting partners with at least a 10 percent chance of having HIV. In the upper classes of these societies, the odds will be much lower. For women from San Sai, or Doi Saket, or Phnom Penh, or the Shan States, they were even higher.

There were three of us in the car: myself, my Thai partner S, and his older sister, Khun O, a teacher. S shares a house with his sister, her husband, and their two pre-teenage children. We were on our way to visit a Buddhist shrine in a limestone cave north of Chiang Mai, a place of pilgrimage. S and Khun O are both devout Christians, members of the Church of Christ in Thailand. They were taking me to the cave, but for them both it was a place of historical, not religious, significance. The conversation was mostly about the U.S. – Khun O had just returned from a school trip with her students. Then we started talking about my work, and about the HIV problem in Thailand. I went into a long monologue on the current challenge: how to protect married women, the difficulty of condom use in marriage, the relative ease of dealing with commercial sex compared to dealing with sex in the home. The car became uncomfortably silent. I sensed I had overstepped the bounds of propriety, and by going on about Thai men's sexual behavior in the abstract, had insulted my friends. It was a relief to get to the cave. Khun O didn't want to join us on the long steep climb into the shrine; S and I went on alone. In the cave, I apologized to S. He stopped me cold:

'No, Chris. My sister couldn't tell you what's happening to her. I was waiting for her to tell you, but she can't. My brother-in-law has taken a minor wife. She thinks he's also going with other women, but she's not sure. She wants him back. We are very against divorce, you know? But she's very afraid. She wants me to go with her to get tested. Maybe in Bangkok. I told her I think he needs to get tested. But how to say?'

10 | THE FLESH TRADE: SEX WORK AND TRAFFICKING IN ASEAN

Trafficking in women consists of the transport, sale and purchase of women for the purpose of prostitution and bonded labor within the country of origin and abroad. This includes a variety of forms and practices under which women live and work in extremely oppressive and/or slave-like conditions. (Cambodian Women's Development Association)

1996

A brothel in Cambodia may offer women and girls trafficked from Cambodia, Thailand, Vietnam, China, or the Philippines. Cambodian women have been trafficked to Singapore, Hong Kong, Malaysia, and Thailand. A brothel in Thailand may have women and girls trafficked from rural Thailand, from Burma, China (Yunnan), Laos, and Cambodia. Japan receives most of its trafficked women and girls from Thailand and the Philippines; as many as 50,000 Thai women may work there. India traffics mainly rural and tribal women and girls, as well as large numbers of Nepalese. Malaysia's sex trade has Cambodian, Thai, and Burmese women, and Indonesians, in addition to Malaysians. Thai women have been found in sexual slavery in California and in Sweden. Vietnamese women have been found trafficked at sea, traded from ship to ship by pirates, homeless and stateless.

This is an industry, and a profitable one, as the African slave trade was profitable in its day. But unlike the legal trafficking of humans in the seventeenth to nineteenth centuries, this form of slavery is untaxed and untariffed. Though illegal, it is low risk compared to trafficking in drugs, tolerated with the right kind of bribes, and offers attractive perks – free access to the merchandise. Trafficking supplies a service – cheap sex – for which there are always buyers. Demand is high in ASEAN countries, and growing as the region's bullish economies grow, as gaps between rich and poor widen, as family and community bonds are transformed by rapid economic and social change.

The sex trade is a relatively small component of the current trade in illegal labor in ASEAN. The Thai Ministry of the Interior estimates in 1996 that there are at least 500,000 illegal workers in Thailand, 375,000 of whom are thought to be Burmese and 100,000 from Laos. NGOs active with illegal workers put the number at closer to 1 million, of whom 750,000 are thought to be Burmese. Sex workers account for only a minority of these persons, 1–5 percent at the most. The majority of laborers work in construction, on road crews, as agricultural migrants, fishermen, loggers, and domestic servants. The same is true for Malaysia, which estimates that there are over 1 million illegal workers in a workforce of only 8 million, and where, again, sex workers would be a tiny minority of these laborers. But trafficking for the commercial sex industry results in human rights abuses on a different scale from most other forms of labor, and it has a much higher mortality rate. Commercial sex is at the heart of Southeast Asia's AIDS catastrophe. And sexual slavery reveals the darkest sides of the countries involved: the status and treatment of women, the power of criminality, the depth and pervasiveness of corruption, what people will do for money.

The Cambodian Women's Development Association estimates that in 1990 there were perhaps 1,500 sex workers and 224 brothel managers in Phnom Penh. A year later, as the country began to open up to the world, and to development aid, there were 6,000 sex workers. After a few months of the United Nations (UNTAC) presence in Cambodia, there were 20,000. Getting this many women into the sex trade requires trafficking, it requires the use of force, and it requires networks to get women from villages to brothels. A United Nations High Commission for Refugees (UNHCR) spokesman put it this way: 'while UNTAC is not responsible for creating Cambodia's current prostitution and trafficking problems, UNTAC's presence facilitated the creation of the apparatus [of trafficking] and the machine has circulated'.

How does the apparatus work?

The trade typically begins in a poor, remote place: an ethnic minority village in Yunnan, an impoverished farming community in northern Thailand, an Akha tribal homestead, or a Shan village caught in the crossfire of the Burmese civil war. About 40 percent of the women in the debt-bonded sex trade in northern Thailand are Shan women and girls. This is one of the better understood trafficking systems, thanks largely to NGO workers in Chiang Mai, one of the destination points for trafficked Shans.

Although abduction happens, as does outright sale of daughters among the poorest of the poor, the trafficking road usually starts with a job offer. A girl is offered work as a waitress, or a maid. Her family usually gets some money. In Thai villages the rate is 5,000–10,000 Baht, in Shan villages somewhat less. This is the start of the debt, and of the bondage. The woman and her family may or may not have an idea what their daughter is headed for, and they may not have many choices.[1] In Burma, the army comes through minority areas frequently in search of porters for their campaigns; two porters for every soldier is standard. Forced porterage in the mountains of Burma is often a death-sentence, and the only way out is to pay. In cash. And so daughters are sent to Thailand in an attempt to protect sons. Among hilltribe peoples such as the Akha and the Hmong, drug debts among fathers have been found to be the commonest reason for the sale of daughters. The networks which supply the heroin know only too well which households are in need of money, and whose daughters are ripe for purchase.

There is a limited number of trafficking routes into Thailand and all require bribes along the way. These are added to the debt. On arrival, the trafficker hands the girl over to a brothel agent. The debt is transferred to the agent. Here she will typically be sold as a 'virgin', whatever her experience. If the trafficker did not violate her already, the agent will. New arrivals are big money; she may not know this, and she may be sold as a 'virgin' 20 or 30 times at the beginning. This is serial rape. The breaking-in process, in which a woman must learn how hopeless her situation is, how little she can do about it, and what sex is. If she refuses, she is raped or beaten, often both. Some escape. Most, in shock, learn the ways of dissociation and forgetting. Then she is trafficked to her destination, a brothel somewhere – it may be in Chiang Mai, or Bangkok, Ranong, Phuket, Hat Yai, or farther afield. Here the debt is doubled.

Most trafficked women and girls arrive at their first workplace owing 10,000–20,000 Baht to the brothel owner. Their wages are further deducted for room and board, for clothes and makeup, sometimes for condoms, always for drugs to treat STDs and for contraception.

After these deductions, a debt-bonded worker usually earns 15 Baht (about 70 cents) for each client she serves. It is with this money that she has to pay off the debt. It can easily take a thousand or more sex acts to pay it off. Many women never make it. Some, particularly tribal women, are innumerate and so cannot keep track of their debts and wages. These girls can get hopelessly mired in debt.

When a woman does, finally, break even, the owner is supposed to start paying her. This is often the time the owner will call the police for a raid. It will cost 3,000 Baht in bribes to get a woman without papers out of jail. The brothel owner will pay this, and the woman will be back in his or her debt. If she refuses, she may be taken to one of the International Detention Centers (IDCs) for illegal immigrants, and from there 're-patriated', usually to the Thai–Burmese border. At the border she will face several options: she can try and get back home, risking Burmese army patrols, arrest, and more rape; or she could talk to the brothel agents, who just happen to be waiting in their pickup trucks. For a fee, they will take her back to another brothel, and she will be in debt again.

Trafficking is slavery of a particularly precarious kind. Most workers trafficked across national boundaries are illegal aliens, and essentially have no rights. Women trafficked into sex work are also criminals in the eyes of the law: the work they do is illegal in itself. They are subject to prosecution in Thailand, Malaysia, Cambodia, Singapore, and China. As many as 10,000 such women come to Thailand each year. And this has increased, not decreased, as education programs have reached the Thai villages that used to supply sex workers. These communities have stopped sending their daughters to the sex trade because HIV has begun to devastate their young people. This has forced traffickers to go farther afield, to find communities – and there are many – where HIV is still a distant rumor, and a few thousand Baht looks like a fortune.

Isn't this illegal? Burma is supposed to be a closed country, with strict limitations on nationals traveling abroad. The plain truth is that a village girl from a remote part of Burma or China does not get to a nightclub in Phnom Penh or Bangkok without the collusion of officials at numerous points in the trafficking process. There are border patrols on both sides, immigration police at check points, and local police on arrival. Khun Anand, former prime minister of Thailand, has pointed to the police and the legal system as the two sectors in Thai society most in need of reform. His observations could be generalized to several neighboring countries. In Cambodia and Burma too, law enforcement is heavily affected by corruption; almost no one expects fairness from the police or justice from the courts, certainly no one without money or influence. Some of the largest sex venues in all three countries are operated by individuals from law enforcement sectors. The police are a national embarrassment to progressive Thais, but remain a powerful, if shadowy, force in society.

Buyers Trafficking is the supply side of the sex industry. What about demand? Who is interested in having sex with a slave? One argument might be that men simply want as much sex as they can get, the terms less important than the release, the sex partner less important than the man's sexual gratification. Brothel sex is not about conversation. If you adhere to biological determinism, several hundred million years of evolution are behind the male drive to spread his DNA as widely as possible. The raising of human infants and children, however, requires long-term emotional stability, the socio-biologists' 'pair bond'. Societies, as Freud argued, have to find ways of balancing the archaic, potent force of sexual desire with the maintenance of socially valued structures: marriage, the family, kinship ties, and now 'sexual health'.

Social solutions to this dilemma vary widely: Muslim Java allows young men the sexual outlet of transvestites; sexual experimentation with male peers is common in many cultures. The modern West, in some settings and social classes at least, tolerates young adult sex before marriage, for boys and, increasingly, for girls. In mainland Southeast Asia, by far the most common sexual outlet for men is the use of sex workers. This was also the case in China before the communist revolution, and it is still true in India, though vigorously denied.

In the Thai case, widespread prostitution has allowed Thai men the valued sexual freedom they enjoy while protecting the majority of unmarried women from sexual experience. Structurally, sex work creates a sub-class of women who fulfill the unmet sexual needs of men, while allowing the society to maintain equally valued female virginity, female monogamy in marriage, and clear lines of inheritance for family wealth. The children a man may father with a prostitute are her problem, not his. Prostitution, sex work as most women and men who do this work prefer, also allows poorly educated women to fulfill their duties in supporting parents. In its modern form it allows low-income families to build the new cement houses that say so much to their communities about status, modernity, and class. It can be, for women who succeed at it, a lucrative form of employment. And it can be slavery.

The demand side of commercial sex in Asia is sharply delineated by class. The play of money and power in the sex trade isn't just between clients and workers, but between wealthy men and poor men. The rich can get fantasy: time with a beautiful and skilled creature who will do their bidding, and who may be making a reasonable living. In studies in Thailand the majority of higher-priced sex workers are divorced women, not trafficked, and often self-employed. Poor men get a raw reality: 30 minutes maximum (usually less) with a frightened trafficked girl on a damp bed. The cheapest sex in Chiang Mai is 40 Baht, less than a bottle of beer. Cambodia and Burma are cheaper still, a woman in upper Burma can be had for 5 Kyat, less than a nickel on the black market. Yet an hour with a Russian woman in Bangkok can cost 3,000 Baht, a 'virgin' up to 10,000. HIV also segregates along class divisions. At a 40-Baht brothel in northern Thailand, up to 20 percent of the women are HIV-infected. In the best massage parlors (some are owned by doctors), less than 2 percent may be positive. For wealthy clients condoms are a trivial expense. For the poorest men, they may substantially increase the cost of sex. This is why Thailand must be applauded for distributing 60 million free condoms per year, and helping to decrease at least the financial barriers to safer sex.

We know less about users of the sex trade in Burma, though commercial sex is generally thought to be less extensive than in Thailand, with the important exception of the gem mines of the Shan and Kachin states, where there are reported to be very large, if covert, numbers of brothels. HIV infection rates among Burma's sex workers in 1994 were high, at an average of perhaps 17 percent across the country, but widespread testing has not been done. It is a much more dangerous undertaking for a Burmese man to visit a sex worker than for a Thai man to do so. Burmese men who visit prostitutes can be charged under the British penal codes of 1886, which make the use of prostitutes equivalent to rape, and carry up to

10-year prison sentences. Careers and reputations can be ruined by such charges. These laws are reportedly rarely enforced, and never against SLORC or its people. But they can be used against enemies of the junta, another component of the mechanics of fear. The effect of these stiff penalties has been to drive commercial sex in Burma deep underground. A friend who recently conducted a health consultation in Burma, which included attempting to look at commercial sex, had this to say:

> There are few formal 'brothels' as such, because these are too easily detected. Instead, men typically contact pimps along certain roads, who then bring girls to their cars. Several men will usually share one woman for a night, with some finding the woman, and others a room to use, which is often more difficult. Each man in the group then has a 'turn' of sex with the sex worker. This informal and fluid system of commercial sex makes education and outreach to the women involved virtually impossible.

Sex is cheap in Burma, but social and health risks are high. A journalist who recently attempted to investigate this phenomenon talked to several sex workers in Rangoon, Mandalay, and Keng Tung. He met a 17-year-old Burmese girl whose mother had sold her to a brothel agent to feed the other children in the family. The girl charged 20 Kyat (about 15 cents) for sex, 100 Kyat for a full night. A full night's work means that the customer is allowed to bring his friends. She had just spent the night with a man and 12 of his friends, each of whom had had intercourse with her twice – 26 acts of penetration in a seven-hour period. For this, she earned less than a dollar.

Given the social 'benefits' of sex work, the release it allows men and the 'protection' prostitution affords the other women in a society, it is striking that so many of the societies that use this mechanism consider sex work so shameful, and that sex workers should be so marginalized. The Cambodians have an expression which captures this attitude: 'If the skirt is torn, do not tear it further', meaning that if a woman has been 'spoiled' she should keep it secret; it should never be made public. Prostitution is illegal in every country in Southeast Asia, including Thailand. Most women involved in the

ASEAN regional sex industry have virtually no rights as workers, and it is they, not owners or managers, who typically suffer harassment from the law. There has been only one successful prosecution of a brothel owner in the 36 years since prostitution became illegal in Thailand. This was the owner of a brothel in Phuket which suffered a disastrous fire, in the wreckage of which were found the bodies of two young girls who had been chained to their beds. The case took eight years to prosecute.

All of these difficulties seem small when HIV enters the picture. It becomes the ultimate occupational hazard. It needn't be so.

In the handful of countries where sex work is legitimate and sex workers have civil and worker's rights, they have impressively low HIV rates. Nevada, the one U.S. state where prostitution is not a crime, has among the lowest HIV rates among sex workers in the U.S. Dutch sex workers are unionized, protected by the law, and empowered to refuse clients who want unsafe sex. HIV infection among these women is unusual. But legalizing (or decriminalizing) sex work means accepting that prostitution is part of your society, that men want it and will use it if available. Moralistic and legalistic approaches, while clear public health failures, have been by far the most common social response to prostitution. There are 49 U.S. states with laws very different from Nevada's. Laws against sex work in Asia, like those in the U.S., have done virtually nothing to protect women, but have worked well to allow considerable profits for criminal trafficking operations, and have, the evidence suggests, facilitated the spread of HIV.

Natural immunity One of the burning questions in current HIV research is natural immunity. There is some evidence that some individuals may be, due to genetic or other factors, resistant to infection with HIV. This has vital implications for vaccine research: if the body already has a way of preventing HIV infection, then we may have a model for designing a vaccine. The first two studies to report this possibility were from Africa, and they were both done in female sex workers. For the heterosexual epidemics of HIV in Africa and Asia, women in the sex trade have become what gay men with multiple partners have been for the homosexual epidemic, a key study population. They represent a core group with extraordinarily high risks for HIV and other sexual pathogens. Their large number of partners and sex acts means that preventive measures can be evaluated much more quickly than among women with only one partner, and fewer sex acts. The sexual acts that happen in brothels, with a woman having multiple different sex partners in a single night, may, however, be biologically very different from sex in the context of marriage. Vaginal flora change. Birth-control practices often differ. Other sexually transmitted diseases are many times more common in sex workers. Sex workers are exposed to men at all stages of HIV infection, including what may be the most infective period of all, the first few months after exposure. Taken together, these differences make sex work an uncertain model for heterosexual transmission of HIV. For studying possible resistance to the virus, however, these same biologic attributes make sex workers ideal.

Two studies of resistance to HIV in Africa have identified small groups of women who, by virtue of their many sex partners, low condom use, and multiple other sexually transmitted diseases, should have become HIV infected, but didn't. One group found six such women in Gambia; the other, 25 in Kenya. Our research group wanted to explore whether this phenomenon was also present in Thai women working in the sex trade. We studied women who also had many partners in a setting where one in ten of their customers may be HIV-positive. We searched our records and identified a handful of women who met these criteria. One was working in a brothel outside a small city, about 40 kilometers from Chiang Mai. The records showed that she had worked in brothels for ten years, since 1986, before the epidemic started, and before condom use was common. We'll call her Khun Noi.

Khun Noi told us she had had, on average, four customers a day, more on festivals and paydays. She usually worked 20–25 days per month, which adds up to more than 10,000 sexual contacts after 9 years. She had had gonorrhea several times a year over this period, syphilis twice, had been treated for recurrent venereal herpes, and had been pregnant twice, but had never become infected with HIV. The odds were wildly against this outcome, and a biologic basis for her lack of infection looked plausible.

I went with the nurses from the provincial STD clinic, women who'd known Khun Noi for several years, to talk with her at the brothel where she worked. We drove outside the town into lush countryside. It was early afternoon, a blazing day in orchard country famous for lychee and mangos. We took a farm road that eventually turned into a dirt track. This track led to a large orchard. We drove perhaps a kilometer through the trees, passing no one. Then we came to a clearing, which was also a parking lot. There was an outdoor beer garden under the trees. About 20 men were quietly drinking beer, sitting on rough plank benches. There was very little conversation, and our arrival seemed to spark little interest. The Mama-San (the word is used by Thais for madam) said that Khun Noi was busy with a client, and would we mind waiting?

I sat on a bench while the nurses chatted with the Mama-San, and watched the scene. Across the benches from where the men were sitting was a kind of outdoor deck. Behind this deck was a string of about ten shacks made of bamboo and tin. Sitting on the deck were perhaps 15 young women. They were watching a Thai soap opera on a portable television. They watched the soap, the men watched them, I watched the men. Occasionally a man would make a gesture to the pimp, a young guy wearing about 12 gold chains, having made his selection. The pimp then told the girl, and she would go to her shack, to be met by the client. After a while, the scene got increasingly bizarre and uncomfortable. The men stared at the women with a kind of flat dull hunger. Country people, farmers and laborers, nonchalant but subdued. Waiting to get laid. The open erotic content of the scene, a country brothel on an ordinary day, made sex impossible not to think about. But it was the lowest common denominator of sex, as bodily function, as commodity, as urge. The women stared at the television with detachment. It was not clear, from their eyes, that they were present at all.

Khun Noi appeared, coming out of one of the shacks behind a man in his fifties, adjusting his trousers as he walked toward his car. She was tall and fair for a Thai, smiling sweetly, and elaborately polite to the nurses, who she called 'older sisters'. They held her hands. There was much laughter all around: it was an utterly natural Thai ladies' conversation.

Khun Noi was an ethnic Shan from a rural part of Thailand's Chiang Rai province. She had come here to help support her family, and had been sending money home, whenever she could, for many years. She had already built her parents a new home. She was 31, and divorced. She had one daughter, who her mother was raising. Although she worked in a fairly cheap rural brothel, she had not been trafficked – she had known what she was getting into; it was common in her home village for women to come south looking for work, and sex work was work. I liked her honesty and her dignity, but I was embarrassed for her in a way the nurses seemed not to be. When she first appeared out of the room I felt a wave of unease, even of shame. I'd been thinking, 'We're sitting here waiting for some guy to come.' It felt uncomfortable too, to be a man in this group of women, when the only reason men came here was for sex. Khun Noi seemed so gracious, so *exposed*, and all the more so for being a bright and personable woman in such a loveless place. I couldn't help but think of the nurses, their husbands, their sons, the knowledge that must be somewhere playing across their minds: he does this too – they all do it.

This is why, since the sex trade is clearly going to continue, sex workers need the protection of the law, access to medical care, and protection from debt-bondage. Sex work does not have to be slavery. ASEAN does not have to tolerate slavery or the corruption that allows slavery to continue. Trafficking will keep HIV flourishing in the region, until there is the political will to do something about it, which means reform of the police, among other large undertakings. Until such reforms come about, HIV will probably continue to have a field day in ASEAN. And women and girls from marginal communities will continue to be trafficked into the short, brutal life of sexual slavery.

Khun Noi, by the way, did agree to be in our research project, but disappeared soon after. It turned out that she was not one of the people with 'resistance' to HIV. She had used condoms consistently with her clients, and never did become infected while working in the brothel in the orchard. She stopped sex work about six months after our meeting, and the nurses told me that she came to visit them about six months after that. She had remarried, and had become HIV-infected through unprotected sex with her new husband. Condoms were for clients, not husbands.

2016: The pledge and beyond

Few issues in HIV have been as hotly contested as sex work and sex trafficking. The organized movements of sex workers in Thailand, but also in Bangladesh, India, Brazil, have long called for decriminalization. For the right to work without police harassment and for recognition of their rights as workers. Sex workers have made the case that they can be essential partners in the fight against trafficking, since they know, often in detail unavailable to others, when a woman or girl is being coerced, trafficked, or otherwise compelled into the work. For many feminists, for many in the human rights world, and for the substantial anti-trafficking and anti-slavery movements that have emerged in recent decades, prostitution is held to be inherently degrading. Calling sex work 'work' reads as an attempt to legitimize sexual slavery. These movements have posited that prostitution inherently leads to trafficking – that the two are inseparable. This may sound like an abstract debate, but it has had far-reaching consequences and involved the largest U.S. program for any single disease in history – PEPFAR.

In 2003, when then President George Bush, established PEPFAR with an initial $15 billion dollar commitment, the HIV world changed. Access to treatment became a reality for millions. PEPFAR also had significant funding for prevention, including condom purchases and HIV testing and counseling. These were the primary foci for both sex workers and gay men in the program. Christian conservatives, who played critical roles in the effort to get Congress to fund the program (and some then serving in Congress and the Bush administration) wanted more. They wanted the U.S. to take a stand against prostitution and against sex trafficking. The result was the inclusion of language, which would become known as the Prostitution Pledge, in the PEPFAR legislation. The Pledge required that any recipient of PEPFAR funds have in place a policy explicitly opposing both prostitution and sex trafficking. Because PEPFAR was established under the State Department, with its head at the rank of ambassador, the legislation which authorized the program made the goal of global eradication of prostitution a part of U.S. foreign policy.

When the policy was announced I was working with a colleague on a large application to PEPFAR. Hopkins needed to have the policy in place. I was tasked with drafting it – a challenge as we wanted to ensure the Hopkins policy would allow for full clinical and prevention services for sex workers – clinical care, counseling, outreach – while still being in compliance with opposing 'prostitution'. There was no difficulty for us (or anyone else applying with whom we were in touch) in taking a stand opposing sex trafficking. Indeed, no one then or now could be found to *not* oppose trafficking – except perhaps traffickers, and they were not seeking HIV funding.

Sex workers and their advocates were inflamed by the pledge, however, and by the deliberate (and in their view inaccurate) conflation of sex work and sex trafficking. The pledge led Brazil to refuse some $40 million dollars in U.S. funding, since Brazil both accepted sex work and included sex worker leaders in its HIV programs.

The public health community was divided as well. While there was and is little debate that sex workers need HIV prevention and treatment services, and that both pragmatism and compassion demanded that they be included in such programs, there was debate about how meaningful the Prostitution Pledge would be on the ground. Would services be interrupted? Would organizations simply stop working with sex workers rather than risk non-compliance with the policy? One aspect of the policy proved to be the most onerous. This was the stipulation that if an organization were to receive any PEPFAR funding, it had to adopt the Prostitution Pledge policy for all its activities, including those funded by other sources. For most non-profits and NGOs, indeed for most players in the global health space, mixed funding is the rule. This eventually led to a constitutional challenge to the law. (Full disclosure, my group wrote a friend of the court brief for one of the plaintiffs challenging the law.) This eventually made its way to the U.S. Circuit Court in New York, where it was, indeed, found to be unconstitutional on First Amendment grounds. Since only U.S. entities have First Amendment (free speech) rights, the victory was a modest one with little implication for the majority of groups serving sex workers.

The struggle continues. SWING, the sex workers union with which we are working in Bangkok and Pattaya, are very clear that they want sex work decriminalized in Thailand. They want workers' rights and the protections and dignity that come from legal recognition. And sex workers, women, men, and transgender continue to have unacceptably high rates of HIV infection – and to be working, technically at least, in an illegal trade.

11 | MILITARY STUDIES

1996

Kai Kawila Royal Thai Army Camp, Chiang Mai, Thailand is the command post of the 33rd Military Circle, for the six provinces which comprise the northern section of the Thai–Burmese border, arguably Thailand's least secure. Huge old rain trees line the service roads through the expansive grounds, past orderly rows of green lorries taller than elephants. You receive crisp salutes as you pass, see army nurses in crisp white, and young men with buzz cuts, green fatigues, and shiny black boots in the fierce heat. The *taharn gain*, the conscripts, look the picture of young male health – athletic, fit, ranging from lean to brutish – marching, doing ground work, shouting out answers to shouted commands. In 1992, every tenth *taharn* in this camp had HIV infection. By 1995, half the beds in the Kai Kawila Army Hospital were reserved for AIDS care – beds that are now nearly always used. The men dying here are very young, many in their early twenties. It takes a visit to the hospital to see how much the image of male vigor displayed on the marching ground is an illusion. This is the army of a smallish country at peace with itself, its neighbors, and the wider world, and yet the death rate here has been higher than in many spectacular battles. To lose a tenth of something is to have it decimated. Decimation is happening here, and not a shot has been fired.

Addressing an audience of high-ranking military officers from a friendly foreign state on the subject of the sexual behavior and drug and alcohol-using activities of their soldiers can be tricky. You have to try to read your listeners' faces, to see what they already know, and how ready they are to face new information, to make tough choices. When I first came to Thailand we had a good deal of information on hand (from an earlier military study) to say that sex with another man raised the risk of a Thai soldier being HIV-positive from one in eight to one in five. This could only mean unprotected anal intercourse, and that the men engaging in it were not using condoms.

We suggested to the officers that we needed to include safer anal sex practices for both homosexuals and heterosexuals in all the military HIV-prevention programs. I know that my voice was steady: I could hear it via the microphone in the cold conference room, but my hands were shaking as I made this proposal. The room, however, was all nods and smiles: 'Yes, we will do that. Next point please.' And they did. During the Clinton debacle over gays in the military, and the subsequent adoption of the 'Don't ask, don't tell' policy, the Thai head of the Joint Chiefs of Staff, General Wimol, was asked if gays would be allowed to serve in the Thai Military. He answered that the Thai Military had always had homosexuals, that many had served with distinction, and that there was no need for a change in policy. Next point please. (What alarms Americans, given the very real threats to peace and stability in the world, is peculiar. We think ourselves practical and Asians mystical, but we respond most powerfully not to information but to symbols: burning flags; sodomy on ships; school prayer; the sexual continence, or lack thereof, of our leaders.)

It seems only natural that HIV should affect armies more than civilians. Most soldiers, obviously, are young men. In Burma the starting age is 15; in Thailand 21. These are young men far from home, family, and friends. They are largely the rural and urban poor, with little or moderate education and limited work experience. Once conscripted, alone and under intense pressure, they seek support from all-male groups, looking for buddies, mates, best friends. We know that this is true from well-conducted studies of the behavior of soldiers, and also from the best war writing: from Hemingway, James Jones, Wilfred Owen, Homer, and Thucydides. Young soldiers drink together; they blow off steam; they go whoring together – as much to be together as to be with a woman. Far from wives and girlfriends, they find cheap brothels close to their bases. The relationship between soldiers and sex workers is as old as war itself; it is for this reason that military medicine has had to concern itself with sexually spread infections in the past, and with HIV now.

Only a handful of pharmaceutical manufacturers are working on HIV vaccines. With few exceptions (currently three), most of the vaccines under development are aimed at only one subtype of HIV: subtype B, present in the U.S., Western Europe, and Australia. A vaccine that worked against this subtype might or might not protect against any of the other subtypes. For the bulk of the potential paying market, this may not matter very much. For most people in the world, who live where other subtypes predominate (Africa, Asia) this limitation may well mean that the HIV vaccines under development will protect neither them nor their children. And, it need hardly be said, these are the great majority of people who are likely to get HIV, though not the B subtype. There is a desperate lack of research activity into the viruses affecting most of the world. This gap has been partly filled by the U.S. Army, and the Walter Reed Army Institute for Research (WRAIR), among others. This is simply because the American soldier is as likely to have sex with a prostitute in Bangkok as in Las Vegas, and is potentially vulnerable to exposure to every HIV subtype known (and some, undoubtedly, as yet unknown). WRAIR has been a leader in HIV research, vaccine research, and vaccine development for the non-B subtypes of HIV. This has also meant that WRAIR has had to establish research partnerships outside the U.S. Its relationship with Thai Army medical researchers goes back 30 years. Thailand has had U.S.-military-supported medical research facilities since then. It is a close, productive relationship, though one not easily grasped by those outside the field. (The most recent success of this collaboration has been the development of a vaccine against hepatitis A, the field trials of which were conducted in Thailand, where the disease is common and a significant problem in facilities like schools and nurseries.)

Many American civilians (and I include myself) have lingering negative associations with our military and its overseas exploits. We associate the medical/ scientific activities of the U.S. military with Agent Orange, napalm and toxic defoliants, and with atmospheric testing of atomic weapons in the presence of uninformed soldiers. We have seen the grainy black and white footage from the Nevada test site, with soldiers lined up in the killing wind. We suspect that we are not told the whole truth about the research activities of the Pentagon. We are not alone in these anxieties: it is still widely believed in the Caribbean and in Africa, as well as among American blacks, for example, that HIV is a U.S. germ-warfare experiment gone awry. (There are several versions of this story, involving an attempt to wipe out the pigs of Castro's Cuba with a CIA-created virus tested first in Haiti, or in Africa. This, interestingly, turned out to have been a KGB disinformation campaign against the Reagan administration, revealed when the U.S.S.R. crumbled and Kremlin documents describing the campaign were declassified.) What is striking about working with the WRAIR group, at least those involved in HIV research – the only ones I know well – is how far their intentions are from such conspiracies. As a group, they are, if anything, more idealistic and impassioned than the civilian research sector. WRAIR's limitations have not, by and large, been a lack of concern or a resistance to working with HIV, as much as budgetary restraints imposed by the Federal Office of Management and Budget (OMB). WRAIR scientists have used sympathetic members of Congress to beef up their HIV budgets for years, performing a rearguard action around the federal bureaucrats whose bottom line has been budget-reduction, not an HIV vaccine that would work against exotic forms of the virus. The political football in this struggle – that of gay men and women serving in the U.S. Armed Forces[1] – has been something of a side issue as far as WRAIR's research program has been concerned.

Because the AIDS epidemic has been so closely connected to homosexuality in the U.S., military and civilian sectors alike have had to confront their own institutional homophobia, and that of Congress, the electorate, and the vocal Christian right. This has been a complex and emotional interaction, fraught with weak, ideological thinking, though it could be argued that the military has done a better job of caring for its infected members than many civilian sectors. Some of this is due to the pioneering work of Dr Robert Redfield, the WRAIR researcher who first described heterosexual transmission of HIV among U.S. servicemen with a history of prostitute use. This was a key contribution: until Redfield's work (it seems incredible now, given what has happened in Africa and Asia, where HIV is overwhelmingly a disease of heterosexuals) being HIV-infected was virtually tantamount to being classed as a hemophiliac, an injecting drug user, or a homosexual man – all grounds for exclusion from the armed forces. After Redfield's landmark paper, one could simply be an unlucky heterosexual. It was General Phil Russell, the head of WRAIR's vaccine division in the mid-1980s, who made another important contribution: he argued that the men and women with HIV in the U.S. armed forces were a potentially valuable group for research on HIV/AIDS. They were eligible for veterans' benefits, and could be followed long-term. Since the military had already mandated regular HIV testing for all members, all HIV-infected personnel could be included in these studies, if they agreed. And agreement has been close to 100 percent, generating some important insights into the long-term survival of people with AIDS while allowing HIV-infected personnel to maintain non-combat duties, dignity, and veterans' benefits. It was a conservative Christian member of the House of Representatives – Dannenmeyer of California – who attempted, against the wishes of the military, to force people with HIV and AIDS out of the armed forces, by means of a pointless, punitive Bill which President Clinton, in an act of calculated cowardice, signed into law in 1996. It is currently being challenged in the courts; the administration clearly knew in advance that this would occur, as it is flagrantly unconstitutional, and violates the Americans with Disabilities Act, made law by President G.H.W. Bush, which includes HIV/AIDS as a disability.[2]

Encouragingly, rates of new HIV infection in the U.S. military have been relatively low, low enough for preventive studies, such as HIV vaccine trials, to have become virtually impossible. So few new infections happen each year that it would take decades, and cost tens of millions of dollars, to find an HIV vaccine using the army as a study population. Enter Thailand, a close U.S. ally, with a large, very high-risk military, high rates of new infection, and a marked eagerness to look for new solutions.

The problem with the Thai Army is that it, too, is a poor population for HIV vaccine studies. Thai conscripts serve only two years, and are difficult to follow thereafter. As they are not volunteers, research on this group is not ethically straightforward. Most crucially, rates of new HIV infection in this group, as we have seen, fell off dramatically once preventive measures had been put in place. By the time an HIV vaccine including antigens against the Thai virus was close to testing, epidemic rates of new infections among Thai soldiers had largely passed. This is why the WRAIR group has been forced to go farther afield, looking at Thai civilians attending STD clinics, at factory workers, at pregnant women, and considering other countries in the region. There have been some questions raised as to why the military should be funding research in civilian sectors. Their mandate, however, has been clear: to protect the American soldier through the development of a preventive vaccine, and there is currently no other way to do this than through expanding the research base.

Some countries, however, are not being considered, most notably Burma. The U.S. military had, until 2016, to its credit (this is a personal opinion) steadfastly refused to deal with various juntas. Burma's army actually reports comparatively low rates of HIV infection – less than 2 percent in 1994 – but these data cannot be taken at face value. The Burmese Army is young: with conscription beginning at 15, it is an army partially composed of children and adolescents, who may not have begun risk behaviors. And, clearly, information on the junta which they themselves are willing to divulge is heavily censored. One study of HIV risks among men in the Burmese military has been reported, though not, as yet, published in full. Risk behaviors were common, and included sex with other men (7.4 percent), extra-marital sex (13 percent), sex with CSWs (37.3 percent), and inconsistent or absent condom use (96.6 percent The prevalence of syphilis was slightly higher than that of HIV, at 2.5 percent. Taken together, these risks and the syphilis finding make the very low reported prevalence of HIV look even less real. There are some differences between the civilian and military health sectors in Burma that may also be of importance. The military has the resources to do a better job of screening blood, to use disposable injection equipment, and to practice safer surgery and medical procedures in general, at least in the cities and at major military installations. What actually occurs is, as always in Burma, unknown. We do know that donations of medical equipment, drugs, and condoms intended for the civilians of Burma have largely been funneled toward the military. And it was the military medical corps which did the behavioral study quoted here, a rare example of the kind of research Burma desperately needs to understand the health and behavior of its people. The Lao military, not surprisingly, is another unknown. One encouraging sign, however, has been a series of discreet meetings between Lao and Thai military medical staff. In a perfect world, the Lao authorities would be able to learn from their Thai neighbors, and initiate prevention soon.

Coda

We have continued to learn from military studies in Thailand about how the Thai HIV epidemic evolves and changes. As HIV rates fell among these serial cohorts of 21-year-olds, a larger proportion of incoming men with HIV had histories of past injecting drug use.

12 | CHASING THE DRAGON: HEROIN AND AIDS

> When a man walks hand in hand with the thirst of craving,
> he will wander from birth to birth, now here, now there, and
> with never an end in sight. (*The Sutta Nipata*)

Dr Ken Nelson has studied the relationships between injecting drug use and HIV since the early days of the epidemic in the U.S. He came to Johns Hopkins from the University of Illinois, after a distinguished career as an infectious-disease physician and epidemiologist, to pursue HIV work. Ken has done medical research in Thailand for more than 20 years, initially on rabies, then on leprosy; he was an American epidemiologist who knew Thailand intimately before HIV arrived. Since then, he has never wavered from an intense focus on mitigating what he knew, by 1991, was going to be a disaster. He brought me to Thailand in 1992, and it was largely through his contacts, and the respect in which he is held by Thai scientists, that we were able to move expeditiously into HIV-prevention research in Chiang Mai.

In Baltimore, Ken had been working for several years with gay men and people who injected drugs, then known as IDU (most injectors in Baltimore use 'speedball', heroin and cocaine in the same syringe). A Johns Hopkins colleague, Dr David Vlahov, had developed the ALIVE study, a large, long-term follow-up program for nearly 3,000 Baltimore drug users. Ken had an elegant idea in the late 1980s, when about 5 percent of IDU per year were becoming newly HIV-infected despite intensive education, counseling, and freely available drug treatment. He thought an essential question could be evaluated among the ALIVE participants. While rates of new HIV infection were falling among gay men, and had fallen to almost zero among hemophiliacs and transfusion recipients in the U.S., inner-city IDU like those in Baltimore continued to be infected at a high, steady rate. One of the few groups of people in the U.S. with ready access to sterile needles are diabetics dependent on insulin. Since diabetics typically need daily injections of insulin, they get standing prescriptions for needles along with their medication. Ken's idea was to compare the HIV rate among diabetic heroin injectors with those who were not diabetic. The result: those with diabetes were strikingly less likely to be HIV-infected than those without the disease. Why? They had legal access to clean needles and knew how to use them. These findings were published in the *Journal of the American Medical Association* in October 1991. The simplicity of this study, and the elegance of its findings, support a conclusion both logical, and, in the American political climate, radical. If IDU had access to clean needles, HIV rates could be reduced.

Narcotics Anonymous (NA), a national support group based on the tradition of Alcoholics Anonymous, defines addiction as an illness. NA maintains that addicts are ill, not criminal. If this is the case, should addicts be treated like other persons in need of clean syringes, such as diabetics, and be allowed prescriptions? This proposition falls under the rubric of harm reduction; while getting off drugs is the ideal in the long term for many who use, harm-reduction strategies seek to reduce those complications of drug use amenable to change, such as HIV infection. Assisting IDU to reduce needle-sharing is harm-reduction, as is needle exchange, another seemingly simple approach to reducing HIV spread among injectors: you offer users new needles in exchange for used ones. Dirty needles are taken out of circulation, and users have less need to share, since the exchange solves their chronic shortage problem. This is practical, simple, effective, and has required a decades-long battle to implement in the U.S.

In the land of 'Just Say No', harm-reduction strategies have proven politically problematic. The arguments against needle-exchange programs have invariably resorted to a handful of unproven, but telling, assumptions: providing needles condones drug use; it promotes drug use; it encourages users to continue using drugs, since using is made safer. None of these assumptions is supported by hard evidence, yet the debate around these simplistic notions has been classically American in its passion and intensity. The evidence suggests, if anything, that addicts in exchange programs are more likely to enter drug treatment, since the exchange programs become points of contact between otherwise isolated addicts and the health care system. Needle exchanges can build trust, open lines of communication, and help build bridges to marginal communities. They can help addicts get into treatment programs. But, like frank sex education in schools, or contraceptive services for sexually active youth, the idea of harm reduction through needle exchange has been seen less as a necessary health intervention than as a moral threat. It took five years for Baltimore to begin a needle-exchange program after the publication of Ken's findings, years in which several thousand people needlessly became infected with HIV. It took an outbreak of HIV and hepatitis C infections among rural whites in Indiana, Kentucky, and West Virginia before Senate and House Republicans finally agreed to federal funding for needle and syringe exchange programs. The ban was lifted in December 2015.

It had been left to activists in the U.S. to mount needle-exchange programs in the great majority of communities where government and public health bodies refused to do so. In many states, such programs were illegal until 2015, underground and under-funded. The same situation existed until 2005 in another country where moralistic (and religious) responses to HIV have made harm reduction a contentious political issue – Malaysia. An underground needle exchange operated in Malaysia on and off for several years. As with public health officials in the U.S., everybody knew it is the right thing to do, and that the scientific evidence is compelling, but harm reduction stood in sharp contrast to the government policy of 'eradication' of drug use.

What did an Islamic nationalist party and the U.S. Democratic and Republican parties have in common? Ideological stances that led to the inability to respond to science with coherent public policy, and vocal fundamentalist minorities who have been successful in compelling governments to shape laws and policies in accordance with their moral and religious dictates. Public health and its practitioners have had mixed results in countering these groups. We have been naive, at best, in thinking that if we did our part well (research, publications, presentations to political bodies), logical outcomes in public policy would follow. But time and again, in Malaysia, and in the U.S., irrational, unsound, and poorly informed policies have been implemented, while those backed by solid data have languished. We have been much less activist in orientation than the anti-scientific fundamentalists, and they have been more successful in shaping policy.

Are there other examples of this? The ban on HIV-infected persons traveling to the U.S. was meant to 'protect' Americans from HIV. It was signed into law when the U.S. already had more than a million cases, more than all of Europe. This ban applied not only to immigration, which might be a more complex issue, and which might actually be enforceable (since physical examinations and blood tests are routinely done on prospective immigrants); just entering the U.S. is illegal for any HIV-positive person. It was this restriction that forced Harvard University to host the 1991 International AIDS Meeting in Amsterdam instead of Boston: an international embarrassment for the Bush administration. George W. Bush began the process of lifting this ban near the end of his presidency. It was finally lifted by President Obama in 2010, after 22 years of pointlessness.

If we look carefully at the pattern of HIV epidemics in Southeast Asia, the first group to undergo the rapid phase of HIV spread in Thailand, Burma, Yunnan, and Malaysia were injecting drug users. In all four cases, needle sharing was the key behavior underlying these bursts. Once several thousand addicts were infected, the spread to non-drug using populations in Thailand and Burma, at least, was rapid and pervasive. This pattern suggests that prevention of early HIV spread among IDU could be crucial for prevention of national epidemics in countries with significant numbers of injecting drug users. This possibility makes harm reduction a priority. Tragically, it has not proven to be any more politically feasible in Asia than in the U.S. Even Thailand, the acknowledged regional leader in prevention, has struggled for decades with implementation of needle and syringe exchange.

1996–1998

The Northern Drug Dependency Treatment Center (NDDTC) is a Thai government facility for the treatment of drug addiction. It is in Mae Rim, a mixed suburban and farming district to the north of Chiang Mai, close to San Sai and Doi Saket, where the widows' group is active. Several kilometers down a country road, beside a Buddhist temple and a small branch of the Ping River, the NDDTC is in an idyllic place. The Director, Dr Jaroon Juttiwutikarn, is a Thai psychiatrist and a specialist in the treatment of substance abuse. The program at NDDTC reflects Dr Jaroon's humane, realistic approach to drug treatment, as well as the Thai government's commitment to funding treatment programs adequately. The basic concept is that of Narcotics Anonymous: addicts are people with an illness who need treatment, not criminals deserving punishment. Admission is voluntary and patients can leave at any time. Heroin addicts are treated with methadone on that problematic tapering dose, opium addicts with tincture of opium, in both cases to relieve the physical symptoms of withdrawal, which can be excruciating. (Detoxification without these treatments is 'cold turkey', an expression derived from the chills of withdrawal, and the pilo-erection – body hair literally standing on end – which gives the withdrawing addict's limbs the look of turkey skin, or gooseflesh.) The program takes three weeks, though addicts can stay longer (up to a year) if they feel the need. In addition to the detox medications, addicts get counseling and health checks; it is a quiet, supportive environment in which to break out of the cycle of addiction. Meditation classes are regularly given by visiting Buddhist monks. There is also Thai traditional therapy. The center's gardens grow Thai medicinal herbs, which are used in a herbal sauna. After the first week of detox in a hospital-like ward, the addicts begin these herbal saunas, and also receive therapeutic massage. These traditional therapies are used to alleviate the physical symptoms of withdrawal, but also to return a sense of well-being and wholeness to people who may have neglected their physical selves for years.

The NDDTC is a beautiful place, and a hopeful one. While treatment failures are common (only about 15 percent of addicts stay permanently drug-free after one admission – the methadone taper is simply too short and doses too low to prevent relapse), and many addicts may be admitted several times for detox before they are finally free, the men and women (and children) who come to NDDTC are treated with dignity, concern, and compassion. Since drug treatment in Laos, Burma, and Malaysia is only cold turkey, and in all three countries is on a criminal, not a medical, model, a significant percentage of patients come from these countries. With the desire to get off drugs, and fear of their own countries' programs, addicts risk arrest to get to Thailand for treatment. The Thai government accepts whoever walks into NDDTC. The first time I went I met a young Canadian girl, half-way through the program, slowly and shakily coming back to life.

While most patients at NDDTC are Thai nationals, only half are ethnic Thais. The other half are tribal people: Hmong, Akha, Lisu,

Lahu, Karen, Yao. The two groups are strikingly different. Nearly all the ethnic Thais are men, most are young, and almost all are heroin dependent, either injectors or men who 'chase the dragon' – heroin smokers. The tribal people are much more heterogeneous: men, women and children are represented. Addicted families come for treatment together. The majority are opium smokers, though heroin use is increasing among some groups. Because opiates are passed through the breast milk of nursing mothers, some of the addicts from these tribal groups are babies. When their mothers stop using, they too go into withdrawal. At NDDTC they are given oral tincture of opium in pediatric doses to ease their suffering. It is an extraordinary sight: tribal women with their babies strapped to their backs walking in groups around the grounds; village women, who are used to meeting at wells, lining up for their daily doses of detox.

The Thais and tribal peoples at NDDTC had very different HIV rates in the late 1990s: about half the Thais were HIV-positive; among the hill tribes, the rate was only about 8 percent. Some of the difference may be due to the Thais being likely to be needle users, and the tribal peoples to be smokers. But some of it may be due to other factors, such as sexual risks. An unknown percentage of the Thai addicts have sold sex to support their habits, a dual risk that is only too common in the West. Will any of Thailand's neighbors follow her lead in the humane treatment of addicts? Burma and Laos, arguably, do not have the resources for treatment centers as well funded as the Thai national ones. Malaysia's program, with its mandatory two years' incarceration, is already many times more expensive, and its success rate no better, if not worse. China also has mandatory drug treatment: it is also cold turkey only, and also has a low success rate. What limits these national responses is largely ideology, rather than science or money. Arguably the most important difference between the Thai approach and that of her neighbors is the voluntary or involuntary nature of programs for drug users. China, Vietnam, Laos, Cambodia, and Malaysia all opted for mandatory detention for drug users. These detention centers shared a lack of real treatment and correspondingly poor outcomes. They also shared brutal regimens of forced and unpaid labor which made them much more like forced labor camps than drug treatment centers. In Vietnam in particular these detention centers became profit-making enterprises built around what can only be called slave labor. In 2016 these centers appear to be returning in force in Vietnam as international donor support for outpatient and community-based programs dries up. Precisely the wrong direction to go in for public health and for human rights.

In the 1990s the Thais had also yet to take two further steps that men like Dr Jaroon know could help reduce the terrible burden of HIV among Thai users. One is needle exchange, which started in Chiang Mai only in 1996; the other is methadone maintenance.

Methadone is a synthetic morphine derivative related to opium, heroin, and morphine. It has similar potentials for dependency as its sister compounds. But it has several features which have long made it the drug of choice for detoxification: it is given orally, so it frees users from needle use; it can manage the opiate craving which drives users back to heroin or opium (scientific evidence suggests methadone may work by saturating the opiate receptors in the brain, thereby reducing the craving for opiates); and it is a legal, prescription drug, which doctors can give to patients. This is something of a historical accident, and there are probably better agents for detox than methadone, but it is legal, so it continues to be used. The standard therapy in Thailand, which is a matter of national policy, is methadone taper: the dose of methadone is tapered off over several months till the addict is 'drug free'. The problem is the craving. Each addict has his or her own level of methadone above which they are craving-free, but below which they start to crave, withdraw, and suffer. Some make it, but many use heroin again, usually in combination with the insufficient methadone dose, to handle the hunger. By the time addicts are tapered completely off methadone, they are often back on their old dose of heroin, and the detox cycle begins all over again. Methadone maintenance accepts that some addicts are not going to lose their craving, at least in the short term, and that going back to heroin use means going back to needle use, and sharing – the spiral of disease risk. Methadone maintenance is another form of harm reduction: let the addicts set their own level of methadone such that they don't need heroin, and let them stay at that dose as long as they need it, to keep them clear of the need for needles, for life, if necessary. (Remember that about half of northern Thai heroin addicts are HIV-infected already, so keeping these men off heroin is essential to protect new addicts from HIV – it is already too late for many long-term users.)

Methadone maintenance was tried once in Bangkok among addicts, in a pilot project done by the Bangkok Metropolitan Authority (BMA) in 1991. While the BMA didn't look at the effect of the therapy on HIV rates, they did look at maintenance in terms of addicts remaining in follow-up and staying off heroin. By those criteria it was an unmitigated success; addicts tapered completely off methadone were much less likely to stay in treatment, and much more likely to go back to heroin use. But, as so often has been the case with AIDS, political considerations delayed the translation of these research findings into public health policy, in this case by at least five years. Why? The Thai Ministry of Social Welfare, which oversees drug treatment programs, refused to change their policy from taper to maintenance. Taper means you are getting people 'off drugs'; it is politically attractive, even if it usually fails. Maintenance means you accept that some people are not going to get free of opiate addiction, but can at least be treated to prevent needle-use relapses. It works, and there is evidence to show that it works, but it is politically 'sensitive', as Dr Jaroon explained to me, too sensitive to implement even in the midst of an epidemic of a new, fatal virus spread through needle sharing.

Why should human frailty be so hard for political bodies to accept? Why are we so tempted by absolutist and simplistic models of human behavior that repeatedly fail to achieve their stated goals? One would think, given the track record of politicians in any country, that they would be the group most eager to embrace forgiveness of human frailty. We look so hard for 'cures', for the magic bullets that will solve complex social and medical problems: a vaccine to protect against HIV, new therapies for AIDS care. But simple steps such as giving users prescriptions for needles, implementing needle exchanges, offering methadone maintenance programs, remain beyond our reach. Compared to the cost and difficulty of AIDS treatment, these are cheap and easy. Preventing HIV spread among addicts might even prevent national HIV epidemics in some countries. But supporting such programs might open a politician to charges of being 'soft' on drugs, and anything is better than that, including being 'soft' on AIDS.

2016

Repeated failures to implement the basics of HIV prevention for people who inject drugs continue to drive HIV epidemics in far too many countries. In 2010, for a special theme issue of *The Lancet* on HIV among people who inject drugs, we reviewed the state of the global state of services for drug users. Just six countries – China, Russia, Ukraine, the U.S., Malaysia, and Vietnam – accounted for about half of all HIV infections among drug injectors worldwide in 2010. Russia had by far the worst prevention record – and the worst outcomes, with a complete ban on methadone or any other substitution therapy, very low rates of needle and syringe access, and extremely low rates of HIV treatment coverage for drug users already living with the virus. Malaysia by 2010 had five years of harm reduction policies in place, and coverage was steadily improving. We reviewed these countries again three years later. The U.S. had not changed (the federal ban on exchanges was still in place) and if anything, Russia had deteriorated. Their steadfast refusal to implement methadone, and the fervor with which they hold to their manifestly failing policies was shown to the world when they annexed Crimea from Ukraine. The Russians stopped Crimea's methadone program *on the first day* of their occupation. Russia's epidemic in 2016 is among the fastest growing in the world. But encouragingly, both Vietnam and Malaysia saw gains in prevention access and success from 2010 to 2013, through implementation of the basics, and through providing drug users living with HIV the treatment they needed to live and thrive.

This is one component of global AIDS we truly do have the science to address. This war in the blood can and is being won. But Russia, and the countries she seeks to influence, are witnessing a self-infected disaster. It is hard to imagine President Putin changing course because public health officials or opinion in the West suggest he is making terrible mistakes. It will be up to the competent professionals Russia has to press for change. We can only hope they succeed, and soon.

For the peoples of Southeast Asia the more proximal threat remains the civil conflict that drags on in the opium poppy cultivation and heroin refining zones of Shan State. These areas are still contested between the Myanmar military, the *Tatmadaw*, and several Shan resistance groups in 2016. *Tatmadaw* troop presence in the Shan hills has increased 40 percent in the past decade, to about 14,000 men. Daw Suu Kyi's NLD government has no authority over the military, as per Than Shwe's 2008 constitution, so there is

13 | TRIBES: THE VIRUS THAT KILLS THE GODS

> [I]t is clear that tribal vulnerability to HIV must be placed within the macro context – national, regional, and global – of changed commercial routes, the entry of urban-based governments and entrepreneurs into the hills, and the migration of hill people into urban centres, as well as the political and economic chaos in neighboring Burma which helps to foster the thriving illicit economy. (Kammerer et al., 'Vulnerability to HIV infection among three hill tribes in northern Thailand', 1995)

The dominant peoples of Southeast Asia have always been low-landers of the irrigated plains and river valleys: the Thais, Burmans, Khmers, Vietnamese. The hills and mountains of the region, tail-end spires of the Himalayan range, have been home to very different peoples. The highland ethnic minorities of Indochina number in the hundreds, and are found in every country of the region. They are a heterogeneous array of peoples, clans, languages, faiths, and ethnicities. These groups include the indigenous headhunting Wa, the stone age 'spirits of the yellow leaves', and the literate Yao, who practice a mystical form of Taoism and venerate the Chinese poet-sage, Lao Tzu. Some, like the nomadic Akha of Yunnan, Burma, and northern Thailand, are animists, though the Akha language is a dialect of Tibetan. Others, like the Hmong of Laos, China, and Vietnam, once had a kingdom of their own, but lost it to Han Chinese, and have been wandering, like the Hebrews, ever since. Relations between highlanders and lowlanders have been a constant theme in the history of the region, often tumultuous, and seldom to the benefit of these tribal peoples.

The great majority of highland communities continue to survive on subsistence agriculture. Slash-and-burn, or swidden, farming techniques are widespread. Prosperity is not. The highlanders lag in education, in health measures such as infant mortality and life expectancy, in literacy, and in political clout. They are a tremendously diverse group in terms of HIV/AIDS risks and rates. Some, like the ethnic Karen in Thailand, have thus far been apparently spared epidemic spread of HIV. Others, like the Wa, the Lahu, and the Kachin of Burma and China, and the Akha in northern Thailand, are likely to be severely affected. Reaching these peoples has not been a priority of most governments in the region. The Shans are still in conflict with the Burmans; the Hmong and Yao in Laos with the lowland Lao; the Mizos, Manipuris, Nagas, and Assamese are in conflict with India, and often with each other. Even where there is peace, the challenges are immense, not only because languages and dialects often isolate the highlanders from majority populations, but also because their understanding of disease and health are often pre-scientific, magical, and unstudied.

The Lahus in Burma are one such group. They are nomadic people from the Tibetan plateau, who have gradually moved south over several centuries. The first Lahu village in Thailand was founded in the 1940s, but they have been in Burma much longer. Burmese is also a Tibeto-Burman language, but is unintelligible to the Lahu. In Burma they have the misfortune to be geographically isolated between the warring Shans, Wa, and the Burmese military, and are themselves divided into several different groups, including the Red and the Black Lahu clans. (These two groups formed a political alliance in the 1990s, the Lahu Democratic Front.) When AIDS education materials first came to the Lahu, these were in the form of pamphlets and posters in Burmese. The pamphlets warned that AIDS was '*nat thi*', meaning incurable. *Nats* are the Burmese folk deities, the local gods. The Lahu interpretation was that AIDS could 'kill *nats*', that this new disease, of which the Burmans were so afraid, killed both men and gods. And this is how HIV was first known among them. What happens to a Lahu woman who comes home after sex work in Thailand, carrying a virus fatal to the local spirits?

As most Lahu in Burma were illiterate in the 1990s, HIV education had to be done through oral media: radio, video, cassettes, talking. The then junta had taken to jamming the uncensored radio broadcasts that once reached the mountains of the Lahu, limiting the effectiveness of this medium for mass education. One solution came from an unexpected quarter: Lahu sex workers in Chiang Mai. With NGO assistance, a group of Lahu women made a series of HIV educational cassettes, and these were distributed through trading networks in the Lahus' remote homeland. These tapes explained not only what HIV was, and how it can be prevented, but also how trafficking works, what a woman can expect if she comes through this route to Thailand, how to use a telephone and what numbers to call if she comes to Thailand and needs help. Because so many tribal groups have had women trafficked to Thailand, such programs, if the groups themselves could accept assistance from 'broken women', could have a significant impact in Burma.

I met one of the Lahu leaders in August 1996, and had a frank discussion about the situation in Burma. His principal concerns were three: injections from untrained practitioners (who he called, charmingly, 'quacks'); heroin use among Lahu men, which he felt was on the increase; and the trafficking of Lahu women and girls. Did he think condom use could be accepted by Lahu men, or at least those men with wives who had been sex workers? Yes, he said, he thought so, but he himself had never seen a condom. What was it, exactly? Did I happen to have one?

We know that the bulk of China's documented HIV cases in the first years of the epidemic were among highland minority peoples; fully 60 percent of the national total of infections by 1995 had been identified in Kachins, Wa, and Dai. In Burma it is clear that highland groups are as heavily affected by HIV as the Burmans – indeed the highest HIV-burdened state in the country is Kachin State – on the mountainous Yunnan border.

In Thailand the first systematic survey of HIV was done among hill-tribe groups: a 1994–1995 survey of nine minorities, carried out by the Thai Red Cross in collaboration with our group. What we found was that HIV rates varied tremendously between groups, from zero cases among the Karen, to 9 percent of all adults among the Shans. The aggregated rate in adults aged 15–45 was 2.1 percent, lower than the Thai rate in the northern region, but higher than the Thai national average. Sexual behavior, social norms, and attitudes toward HIV all varied just as strikingly; these groups are as different from each other as the Irish are from the Yoruba. But one thing did not differ greatly, and this was the risk factor associated with being HIV-positive. There was really only one risk, and it superseded ethnicity: for women, having been a worker in the sex industry; for men, having been a patron. In our study at least, tribal people with HIV were those who had been touched by the sex trade in the lowlands. We found HIV-infected women in seven of the nine ethnic groups studied, but infected men in only three of the nine. The two groups where no cases were found, the Karen and the Pa-long, police their own communities and do not allow trafficking. Several Karen communities are known to shoot brothel traffickers on sight. This may not be a prevention strategy that one would like to see spread, but it cannot be called a failure.

My Thai colleagues and I have presented the findings you have just read many times in Thailand, to academic audiences, medical groups, and the government. Each time we've done so the results have been met with disbelief. The usual assumption is that the tribal groups have much higher rates than the Thais, due to their habits of 'free sex', their loose morals, poor hygiene, and heavy heroin use. That the major risk for HIV among minority peoples should be the Thai sex industry seems incredible to Thai audiences. But the evidence is fairly compelling. If local spread were the root cause, we would expect to see what is found in most other communities: either equal rates among men and women, or higher rates among men – not four ethnic groups where all HIV-positives were women and none men. But the highlanders are a classic example of the 'other', the 'outsider', to lowland majorities, and HIV comes from the other, not the self.

HIV prevention for these communities in Thailand is clearly going to require a focus on trafficking. In China, heroin use will be key. For the ethnic minorities in Burma, both heroin use and trafficking are going to have to be addressed, and both will be extraordinarily difficult to remedy. For the hill tribes in Burma, the prognosis is painfully poor. Of the highlanders in Vietnam, Laos, and Cambodia, little can be said as so little is known. The one exception, perhaps, is the Hmong of Laos, who have a long, complex history of exchange with the outside world, who have been known, even if they are now abandoned and forgotten.

Diaspora: the fate of the Hmong

The domino theory of communist expansion has been fairly thoroughly discredited. It now seems as dated and wrong-headed as the Hollywood blacklist, or the 'red' in Red China. The media, with their seemingly unconscious Western bias, routinely talk about the 'fall of communism'. We find ourselves saying 'now that the Cold War is over', just as we stumble over leaving out 'the' when we say Ukraine. But while the Czechs race toward Europe and the many new -stans to Islam, China, Vietnam, and Laos are still ruled by communist politburos. The men who led the communist revolutions of these neighbors are very much in power. The Hmong people of Laos really were a domino that fell to the communists. They paid the heaviest price you can pay for their resistance to the Viet Cong-supported takeover of Laos: defeat, impoverishment, loss of their native lands, slaughter, and exile.

The Hmong are a proud, fierce people. Accounts by the French and Americans who fought with them are strikingly consistent in their respect for these small, tough, mountain people. It took nine years of war and the invasion of over 70,000 Vietnamese troops to drive the Hmong off their mountains in Laos, so fierce was their resistance. More than 100,000 Hmong from those mountains have been resettled in the U.S., where the rich, ancient Hmong tribal culture is a poor preparation for immigrant success. Self-sufficient people of the limestone crags, slash-and-burn farmers, hunters and trappers, they now must survive on the outskirts of Los Angeles, San Diego, and Minneapolis.

No one knows how many thousands of Hmong were killed during the long wars in which they fought beside two losers, the French and the Americans. (The French called them *montagnards*, and used them as scouts. The U.S. CIA used them as a proxy army against Vietnam.) The real slaughter came later, after the capture of Vientiane, when the communists took their revenge with the simple slogan, 'wipe them out'. Perhaps half the Hmong population was killed in the ensuing genocide (there is no other word). Those who managed to escape to Thailand faced lives of poverty and despair in crowded camps. Unused to lowland conditions, to overcrowding and inactivity, many died. The lucky families got out, to the U.S., Australia, or France. The rest remained in Thailand until 1993, when the Thais initiated a policy of forced repatriation to Laos. More than 16,000 have been sent back since then. This late chapter in the saga of the Hmong was almost totally ignored by the world's media.

The UN High Commissioner for Refugees was supposed to be overseeing the Hmong *refoulement*, but rights monitors were not given permission to go beyond Vientiane, and that is not where the Hmong were. It was not at all clear what was happening in the mountainous interior of Laos. The people who slaughtered the Hmong are still in power. I had been told that Laos was quiet, and it was portrayed that way in the media. In Vientiane we heard rumors of fighting and insurgency in the interior, but these were unsubstantiated.

On a river journey from the Thai border to Luang Prabang in 1996, we passed several new villages of Hmong recently sent back to Laos. These riverine areas were never Hmong lands in the past. Their homeland is the mountains surrounding the Plain of Jars, the scene of their great defeat. In Luang Prabang itself, the Hmong were nowhere to be seen. On the last day of my stay I met two men on the street who had the classic stocky build and broad, high foreheads of the Hmong. The older man, about 30, asked me in English where I was from. When I said 'America' his face lit up, and so I knew he was Hmong, not Lao. We went for a walk; he was furtive, checking all directions as we went. I asked him how things were for him, now, in Laos.

'It is very bad for the Hmong. I cannot work, we have no way to make a living. Two years ago my family and I were sent back here from Chiang Khong, in Thailand. We did not like Thailand but at least we were safe there. My family is in the mountains now, some days' walking from here. I will take you if you want to see. This Lao government is very bad to us. We are forced to fight again.'

'Is there fighting now?'

'Yes, fighting. But we are alone. No one is with us.'

I promised him I would try and return, would talk to journalist friends, to try and generate some interest in their plight. He gave me his name and address and we said goodbye.

That night, when I came back from dinner, he and several more Hmong were waiting outside the hotel gate. They wanted to share my room, as they had no place to stay. But it seemed unsafe for them; the hotel was government-run; officials from Vientiane were staying there, and five Hmong men would be fairly obvious in my single room. We walked through the night streets together for a while. Their belief in the Americans was moving, but also tragic.

How was I to tell them that we were most unlikely to come back and assist with their current troubles?

Soon after this meeting, a young Lao man, keeping a safe distance but always there, followed me wherever I went. Having spoken with my new Hmong friends, I had acquired a tail. This fellow appeared at the airport the next morning, as I got ready to fly back to Huai Sai on a Lao Aviation biplane. He managed to sit next to me on the flight, and I noticed he was carrying no luggage, in stark contrast to all the other Laos, who were loaded with bags, stacks of French bread, whole banana bunches. He was met by three army officers on the tarmac; I made one more round of police checks, and was allowed to leave. A bad Graham Greene sequence, but also a reminder of how tightly controlled and mistrusted the Hmong remain. I contacted several journalists on my return to Thailand. Two or three had already heard that there was fighting again between the Hmong and the Lao, but no one was interested in covering the story. 'It's just a drug war', said one, 'nothing political is happening there.' The Hmong in Laos had always grown opium for medicinal use, and for the aches and pains of old age, for which it was especially reserved. Because of Laos' isolation, high mountains, and the unnavigable stretches of the Mekong as it moves south through the country, the French saw little hope of developing Laos for the lucrative plantations they had already established in Cochin. Their policy in Laos was to impose a yearly 'head tax' on all adults, and to collect this in silver. The Hmong had nothing to sell but opium, and this the French accepted. So began the long history of the Hmong as opium growers.

The Hmong in Thailand were also opium farmers, until the Thai government policy of crop substitution reached their highland homes. Some have succeeded in growing cut flowers or fruit, and in trading. But the loss of opium revenues has had an economic impact, and an impact on HIV as well. There is some evidence that as opium became unavailable for the Hmong, users switched to chasing the dragon or injecting heroin. Striking correlations have been shown by researchers at Chiang Mai University, and by the Center for AIDS Prevention Studies (CAPS) in San Francisco, of the simultaneous rise in heroin use with the decline in opium smoking. Opium the Hmong grew, heroin they must buy. And so the trafficking of Hmong girls increased as well, as addicted fathers sold their daughters for heroin money. The Hmong in Thailand now have a significant HIV problem (Vietnam is an unknown, as is China, where there are 5 million Hmong).

If it is true that suffering is a magnet for HIV, that it is drawn to add yet another burden to people who already have many, this latest twist in the fate of the Hmong only makes sense.

14 | THE DISPLACED: MIGRANTS, REFUGEES, IDPs, AND HIV

> 'This is not our home, but this is where we have to live', said Daw Htoot Hsan, 62. 'Our country is not at peace and we have to make the best of it. But we still want to go home.' (Kachin internally displaced woman, Myanmar, *Myanmar Times*, June 9, 2015)

The world is on the move. Forced or willing, alone or with whole clans, there are more human beings displaced from home and homeland in 2016 than ever before. The Syrian horror and the wider conflict in the Middle East are at the heart of a vast new diaspora. But so too are multiple, no less troubling, drivers of displacement worldwide. In Africa, the authoritarian regime in Eritrea, the Somali failed state, the bloody birth of South Sudan have all led to mass displacement and migration. In the Americas, the war on drugs and subsequent gang violence have left young Central Americans with few options but to flee their homelands or face the gangs – or be forced to join them. In Asia broadly, and in Southeast Asia in particular, much of the migration is for work. Regional economies, the Philippines, Thailand, Myanmar, rely on remittances from countrymen laboring abroad – and on cheap migrant labor at home. Thais work in the Gulf and in Israel. Burmese, Lao, and Khmers work in Thailand. Indonesians in the hundreds of thousands work in Malaysia. Burmese Rohingya work in Malaysia's dirtiest jobs – while Myanmar claims the Rohingya, in Burma for centuries, are illegal aliens from a place which no longer exists as such, Bengal. All are at risk for what are called the three 'D's of undocumented migrant labor; dirty, dangerous, degrading.

Some of these displaced people come from HIV endemic or epidemic countries, like the 2 million or more Zimbabweans who have been forced to flee Mugabe's corrupt and despotic rule. Others like the Syrians, have fled a country where HIV was rare, but are now facing contexts of rising risks – where women and girls are much more likely to be sexually exploited, where survival sex, vanishingly rare in what was a highly educated and conservative society, is on the rise in this catastrophic period. Among the millions of displaced Afghans during their years in Iran and Pakistan, bored and frustrated young men were much more likely to initiate drug use, and heroin injection. This too is a risk for the displaced of the Middle East.

LGBTQ migrants and refugees are in the global mix as well – Ugandans and Syrians, Kazaks, Nigerians, Russians, and Jamaicans, forced to flee homophobic violence from anti-gay regimes or the police, but also from communities, and painfully enough, sometimes from their own families. President Obama's lifting of the visa ban on HIV-positive persons coming to the U.S. opened a tightly closed door for those living with HIV. Secretary Hillary Clinton's policy shift toward LGBT rights, and Secretary John Kerry's directive that U.S. embassies and consulates worldwide include discrimination based on sexual orientation and gender identity as grounds for seeking asylum, opened another. The election of Donald Trump to the U.S. presidency may well shut down this vital escape route for persecuted gay and trans people. Time will tell.

The displaced are enormously medically underserved in much of the world. While those with formal refugee status (generally granted by the UN and largely for people in designated refugee camps or other kinds of settlements) are meant to have access to a basic minimum of health, nutrition, and sanitation services, such refugees are a minority of the displaced. In the Middle East, in places like Colombia, South Sudan, DR Congo, and Myanmar, many more are internally displaced persons, IDPs, still within their home countries but not in their homes. Many have little access to care. What aid does reach them can be limited by hostile governments, conflict, basic logistics. Those crossing borders without documentation, without work permits or visas, are often unable to access health care in the countries where they labor. Rural migrants to China's vast cities may be denied health care where they work – with rights of access tied to home addresses in distant provinces – and with little or no ability to change official residence status. Persons in all these contexts who have HIV infection may face treatment interruptions when they leave home. And, of course, many countries screen migrant workers for HIV – this is ubiquitous across the Gulf states – and deport any

HIV-infected workers they find. Taken together, the displaced may constitute one of the largest populations unreached by HIV services. Since untreated HIV infection is infectious HIV infection, the lack of HIV treatment poses threats to the lives of these vulnerable individuals and may also undermine HIV control.

Thailand, to her credit, has tried to address these issues for people living with HIV in the kingdom and who are not Thai. They have a registration system for migrant workers, a policy of former Prime Minister Thaksin's, which has given some legal status to over half a million workers. Through this registration, migrant workers can access the Thai public health system (the famous '30 Baht' scheme – another Thaksin policy) and get up to one year of antiretroviral therapy. After that, they need to seek HIV care in their home countries. A bridging measure, essentially, but one with more humanity than is found in many other countries in the region.

Mae Sot

Sixty years of ethnic conflict in Burma/Myanmar have displaced millions of ethnic minority peoples within and beyond this troubled country. In 2016, the displacement continues, though some of the affected communities have changed. Some, like the Karen and Karenni refugees of eastern Burma, who have been in camps in Thailand for up to three generations, are now starting to go home. Footage of the first few busloads to return appeared on Facebook in late October 2016. Anxious families waving out the windows of blue buses. Saying goodbye to camps many had been born in. Yet mass displacement continues just a few hundred kilometers to the north, in Kachin State where five years of fighting have displaced over 100,000 Kachin civilians, and where more than 35,000 languish in IDP camps – vulnerable to shelling from the military, over which the new NLD government has been unable to exercise control.

I first went into Eastern Burma's zones of conflict and displacement before I'd ever been to Burma proper. In 1994, a malaria outbreak struck the student army then resisting the SLORC regime from a jungle base on the Salween River. The All Burma Students Democratic Front, the ABSDF, was an idealistic group of university students – the best and brightest of Burma. They had joined or led the student protests of 1988, which triggered the wider popular uprising. When the military cracked down, many were killed. Some who fled to the jungles to the east of the country joined together and formed a student army to resist the regime. The forested hills and mountains of the Salween drainage where they had set up headquarters were malaria country – heavily endemic for *Plasmodium falciparum*, the most serious form of malaria, which can cause the high fevers and anemia common to all forms of the disease (there are four) but also both cerebral malaria and black water fever, often fatal if untreated. The indigenous Karen and Karenni peoples of this region live with malaria, in that time little treated, and they suffered with it – losing babies and small children, pregnant woman, some adults. But they also built levels of tolerance if they survived recurrent bouts. The students were mostly from urban Burma – they had never had to sleep out in the jungles until they'd fled Rangoon and Mandalay in fear for their lives. Malaria hit them hard. I'd been asked to bring malaria medications since the student's supply had been looted in a recent Burma Army raid – the soldiers of the regime were suffering from malaria too, and they too were short on anti-malarial drugs.

Conflicts can simmer and erupt weirdly close to places at peace. The drive from Chiang Mai to the Burmese border crossing is just a few hours. And in those hours, you can go from busy market towns full of goods, quiet farms, to forest tracks threatened with snipers, paths strewn with landmines, young men in arms on both sides of contested hills. We drove to the Thai–Burma border with a rental jeep full of malaria medication. Much of the border here in the Thai province of Mae Hong Sorn, is the Salween. One of Asia's last undammed rivers, the Salween comes rushing from glacial headwaters on the Tibetan Plateau. Even on the hottest days of *ro doo rawn*, the hot season in Thailand, the gray waters of the Salween are icy cold. Both the Burmese and the Thais fear this river (neither people can commonly swim) which they say has a malevolent spirit which pulls people under its swirls and eddies. We were met at the small Salween river port of Mae Sam Lap by a group of students who were to escort us to Dawgwin, the student camp about three hours upriver. They traveled with a long-nosed boat, a slender motorized craft that is easily tipped. I have a deep lifelong aversion to guns of any kind. But we had to ride with armed men at both ends of the long-nose – their eyes fixed on the Burmese bank of the river, since snipers had been active there in recent weeks.

In the event, we made it to the student camp without incident. The boxes of meds were quickly unloaded and on their way to the makeshift clinic before we walked up from the bank to the camp. It wasn't hard to gauge the severity of the outbreak – young men and women could be seen lying on hammocks or benches wrapped in piles of blankets, shivering with the awful rigors of malaria. The student leader, a young physician from Mandalay, greeted us with a weary smile. He too had been ill. He would become a good friend and a valued interpreter of the complex politics of his country. He was leading his several thousand student soldiers in an alliance with the Karen – the indigenous people of the rainforests of eastern Burma, who were fighting one of Asia's longest insurgencies, against Burma military rule over their lands. The Karen called their land *Kawthoole*. They had been fighting for it since 1948.

For the next several years I would spend increasing amounts of time along this border, on humanitarian missions, visiting the crowded camps where some 140,000 people, many the families of Karen resistance fighters, sheltered on the Thai side of the border. In 2000 several donors to the relief and health efforts along the border requested a formal evaluation of the health services. I agreed to design and conduct the evaluation, along with my husband Mike, a nurse practitioner, who was to lead the evaluation of clinical services.

Our base for the project was the center of health care for the peoples of eastern Burma, the Mae Tao Clinic built and run by Dr Cynthia Maung. Herself a displaced Karen from Burma, she was one of the many forced to flee in the aftermath of the 1988 uprising. Dr Cynthia started out providing emergency care in a shed to students and others wounded in the uprising or its aftermath. Under her steady leadership Mae Tao grew over the years into a hospital, a center for health training, a community health program, indeed, a health care system, with satellite clinics and mobile teams working across eastern Burma's conflict zones. Mae Tao served the Burmese diaspora on both sides of the border. The more than a million migrants in Thailand, laboring outside the camps and with no access to health care and the internally displaced in eastern Burma, reached through mobile teams, called Backpack Medics. Our evaluation of this health system uncovered some areas where work was needed. One was on health information systems – there had been no systematic effort to categorize the burden of diseases, the causes of deaths, among the peoples of this heavily militarized region. Working with Dr Cynthia, with teams of Backpack Medics, the Karen Department of Health and Welfare, and with a great group of physicians from UCLA's Global Health Access Program, GHAP, we began a series of collaborative efforts to better measure health, assess the interactions of health and human rights, and, eventually, to try to intervene on some of the major killers.

Malaria was the single greatest threat – accounting for about 45 percent of all adult and child deaths – an extraordinary burden. Contrary to the thinking that this was a 'low intensity' civil conflict, we found a huge gender gap among men and women of fighting age. The men were missing in enough numbers to distort the population structure. When we looked at the numbers in comparison to other civil conflicts, only communities in Afghanistan and Angola during their decades of conflict had comparable numbers. This conflict, though largely unknown to the wider world, was far from low intensity. Landmines injuries and deaths were off the charts as well – another symptom of the depth of the losses. (In 2016 Burma ranks third worldwide in landmine injuries and deaths, behind Colombia and Afghanistan, and large-scale demining efforts have yet to begin.) Complications of labor and delivery were significant killers of mothers and their infants. So too were diarrheal diseases, especially among children under five, and among adults who'd been forced into serving as porters for the military. The *Tatmadaw* forces were taking young men (and sometimes older men and women) as forced laborers to carry their supplies and equipment over the forested hills. Underfed, overworked, beaten, and forced to drink water from streams and ditches, these porters were at great risk of sickness and death.

Some of the communities the programs worked with were relatively stable – under Karen control or near the border. Others, in more contested areas or under Burmese Army control, were internally displaced communities in hiding – on the run because of village burnings, fighting, or because of the predations of the soldiers for portering, forced labor for road crews.

The border programs could do little to address HIV in these zones. The populations were mobile, sometimes in hiding, and the kinds of long-term monitoring and care that are required to treat HIV were just not available. Even testing and counseling proved problematic. There was little way to protect confidentiality – many of the health workers were people from the same small communities. Since malaria was a major killer, and one which could be addressed, the focus had to be on improving malaria prevention (using insecticide impregnated bednets), rapid diagnostics, and treatment with anti-malarials. Most of the mobile medics visiting these communities were young men (after the rape of a young woman medic by regime soldiers) and in Karen traditional culture it was not appropriate for young men to ask unrelated women about sexual risks – so these were impossible to ascertain.

The Mae Tao clinic did have a program prevention of mother-to-child transmission of HIV, including screening all pregnant women, and working with the local Thai hospital to ensure women who were infected got services to prevent transmission. Data from that program suggested about 2 percent of pregnant women attending the clinic had HIV infection in 2005, roughly similar to Thailand's rate at the time. But almost no one in eastern Burma was able to access HIV treatment in these years. When patients with AIDS did appear at Mae Tao clinic they were usually in extremis – too sick to walk or to stand. AIDS patients in Thailand were already having their Lazarus moments at this time, but for the displaced of the borderlands this was years away. This hard truth persisted for many years.[1] When we think about displaced communities, and the services they need which can be delivered through simple approaches like mobile medical teams, the limitations on HIV care are stark. Simple as HIV treatment has become, it still requires accurate diagnoses, long-term follow up, clinical monitoring, retention. When populations were as mobile as the ones in eastern Burma, the logistics made HIV care, like treatment of chronic diseases or cancer, a bridge too far.[2]

15 | OTHER GENDERS: *KATOEYS, WARIA, HINJRAS, TOMS,* AND *DEES*

The great mother created three beings, the first man, the first woman, and the first *katoey*. (Lanna Thai origin story)

Man or woman, boy or girl, male or female, straight, gay, or bisexual – these categories of sex, gender, and sexual preference seem straightforward. They make biological sense. They come out of our world and have shaped it, from Adam and Eve to the nuclear family. What it means to be a man may vary across time, place, and culture; what it means to be male we think of as much less varied – it's the birds and the bees ... until you look at bees for a while, and realize that their genders are not so simple. Queens are made and not born (she who is fed royal jelly develops the great reproductive reservoir). Gender, for bees, is a task category, determined by the needs of the hive as much as by individual biology. Birds are not so straightforward, either. A subset of male ostriches prefers to live with other males, developing elaborate dances done with flexible necks and ticklish tails; some will kill any ostrich chicks they see. Herring gulls have high rates of female–female coupling. Lesbian gulls mate for life (does this sound familiar?) and lay double batch after double batch of unfertilized eggs.

What does it say of our clean dichotomies of sex that some cultures think there are three genders? Or that everyone is bisexual, or that no one is? Or that there are two kinds of women, one female and one male, but only one kind of male, who can have sex with both kinds of women and still be straight? Adam and Eve, and ... Eve's half-sister? There are three genders in traditional Thai culture: men, women, and *katoey*, the last category being persons born with male bodies, who perceive themselves (and are perceived by others) as female. They take on female dress, speak the female dialect, live from childhood through life as women, though of a special kind.

The origin story of the northern Thais serves as their version of *Genesis*.

> The great mother created three beings, the first man, the first woman, and the first *katoey*. The *katoey* was jealous of first man's love for his wife, and killed her to have first man for his own. Because the *katoey* was also male, the marriage with first man was childless. The great mother killed them both and started again, creating second man, second woman, and second *katoey*. This time the second *katoey* felt his male energy, and was jealous of the man. He killed him, but wanted to live with the second woman as a sister, not a wife. Again the union was childless and again the great mother killed them both. When she created third man, third woman, and third *katoey*, she pulled the third *katoey* aside and told him that he must let the man and woman live together and produce children so that creation could go on. The *katoey* would have a special role, but had to accept this marriage. The *katoey* agreed, and the Lanna people came into being, filling the valley with their offspring.

It is a strange story to Western ears. The *katoey* is an ambiguous and potent figure, who must be compelled to make peace with both men and women so that the world can be populated. (S)he is something of a wild card, a dangerous element, but creation is not complete without her/him. Each time the genders are made anew, there are three.

When we started interviewing soldiers in the Thai Army about sex with other men, we got a somewhat low response rate; 3.7 percent said they'd had sex with another man at least once in their lives. This seemed low, not only because Thais tend to be candid about sex, given the right interview environment, but because other groups had already reported rates as high as 14 percent, also among Thai soldiers. One of our interviewers, a young Thai man from Chiang Mai, and a native dialect speaker, suggested that our questions were the problem. We were asking, 'Have you ever had sex with another man?' using the Thai word *puchai*, man. Why should that be confusing? Because man does not include *katoey*. We then asked, 'Have you ever had sex with another man, or with a *katoey*?' The response rate more than doubled. The problem was that there really are three genders in northern Thai culture, and we had asked about only two of them.

What is a *katoey*? Biologically speaking, she is a normal male, as far as modern science goes. The word itself is thought to come from archaic Khmer: '*ka*' is derived from the word for person, '*toey*' from a word signifying 'other', or 'stranger', literally, another kind of person. Not far, perhaps, from the English 'queer'. Are *katoeys*, the often beautiful and always ultra-feminine Thai ladies (most with penises and scrotums) born or made? Male or female? Gay or straight? My friend, the lovely Nadia from Pattaya, can answer all of these questions without skipping a beat. She was born the way she is. She is a *katoey*, which means being a special kind of woman, not a man. She has *jai ying*, a woman's heart. And she is *100 percent* straight: gay men do not interest Nadia. Having an affair with another *katoey* would be either incest or lesbianism, and she is into neither. She wants a real man. And, in Thai culture at least, real men want her.

In the army data, several of the men who said they had had sex with *katoeys* did not have sex with anyone else, not other 'men' or other 'women', just *katoey*. A fourth gender? But most of the men who'd been with *katoeys* also reported many other partners: wives, girlfriends, female sex workers. In fact, these men (who we might be tempted to call 'bisexual', although they certainly wouldn't be) had, on average, more female partners than the men who had only female partners. When I pointed out this finding (it came from an analysis I was doing and I did not, at first, believe it, much less understand it) to a Thai colleague, he said 'Oh yes. They are just *nak tio*', a rough translation of which would be 'hard-core party animals'. And they had the HIV rates to show it: 18 percent were infected by the age of 21, as opposed to 12 percent of men who had sex only with women.

Thai men like *katoey* for several reasons. In purely erotic terms, they will do things, like oral sex, that Thai women, especially social equals like wives, are taught to think of as dirty. They are described as 'tight' and 'dry', references to the muscular anal sphincter. But like good Thai women, they will support a man, work to put food on his table, and tolerate infidelity with other women. One Thai friend told me that his mother was very upset when he had a young male lover – such boys cost money; they want nice clothes; they make demands. She was greatly relieved when he brought home a *katoey*, because, as she said, 'The *katoey* will take care of you, not the other way around' – Thai practicality at its best.

In traditional times the *katoey* had a lot of work to do to keep up feminine appearances: shaving, make-up, false breasts, concealing male genitalia, should a partner want this hidden. They did not, like the *hinjras* of India, self-castrate. Now, of course, there are female hormones; breast, lip and buttock implants; plastic surgery to reduce the ears or the nose; and, finally, castration and vaginoplasty – the surgical creation of female genitals out of male ones. This process – transsexual surgery, or gender 're-assignment' – is reserved for very particular cases in the West, cases of what we call true transsexualism. This is a relatively uncommon condition, characterized by lifelong, persistently held beliefs and feelings of having been born in the wrong body. In the U.S. and Europe, surgeons will operate only after a person has had a minimum (in the U.S., typically two years) of psychological counseling to be sure that this is what they want. Often, two independent psychiatric evaluations are further required. This is to ensure that the gender-identity issue is the real one, and that there is not some other, underlying pathology which would drive a man to want to be castrated, or a woman to want to have bilateral mastectomies, a hysterectomy, and to go through puberty again.

In Thailand, all that is needed is the money. Transsexual surgery is done on demand, and many *katoey* have undertaken it. Are they the same as what we call 'transsexuals'? Or are they really a second form of woman choosing to become the first kind, the one without a penis? Nadia, who has had the surgery, is again clear on this issue, which I raised with her one drunken evening in Bangkok: she is still a *katoey*, but a more complete one.

Many *katoey*, particularly those who sell sex for a living (estimated to be 75 percent of the community in 2016, according to *Sisters*, the transgender support group based in Pattaya) don't have gender affirming surgery, or defer it till their sex work career is done. Why? Many men want a woman with a penis. The transwomen also titrate their female hormone doses so they can maintain erections – since many male clients want to be penetrated by a woman. It does take all kinds.

Do these traditions survive, or did they ever exist, elsewhere? The Laos, being first cousins of the Thai, also have *katoey*. The identical term is used. Laotian attitudes appear to be similar to Thai ones, although the unanimous sentiment (in Vientiane and Luang Prabang) is that Thai *katoey* are more beautiful because they can afford hormones – Lao *katoey* still look more like men in skirts. (Nadia's mother is Lao; she loves her son like the good daughter she's become.) Burma has another ancient and still vibrant tradition: the *nat pwe* performers. The 37 *nats* of Burmese tradition are semi-divine beings, usually humans who met terrible deaths in the historical past, worshipped through shamanic trance-like ceremonies. *Nat pwes* are the festivals held to honor these deities. The priests and priestesses of this unique Burmese cult 'marry' the *nats* they serve, with male priests becoming 'wives'. When this mystic marriage has occurred, the *nat* priest takes on female clothing, speech, and behavior, becoming, as it were, a kind of holy drag queen. Their fantastic costumes, elaborate face paint, and wild dancing style can only be described as high camp. While many *nat* priests and worshipers are not gay, the great *nat pwe* festivals serve as Burma's gay and transvestite gatherings. The largest one, at sacred Mount Popa, is said to attract 20,000 gay Burmese, and must be one of the world's singular parties. During the pro-democracy uprising of 1988, Burma's transvestites and gays had their own section marching through the streets of Rangoon. They were active participants in the struggle against the military, and there is video footage of their liberating parade past the waiting guns.

The first Burmese modern novel to be nominated for a major literary prize, Nu Nu Yi's 2008 *Smile as They Bow*, is about an aging *Nat Pwe* medium and the impoverished young man he loves. Salacious, touching, the book is also subtle political satire which skewers the wealthy society ladies (the wives of generals and cronies) who pay for the medium's divinations. *Smile as They Bow* is matter-of-fact about the gender-bending at its heart, and about the love story it portrays.

The *waria* of Indonesia are another transgender group in the region, one which serves an interesting role in Muslim-dominated Java. *Waria* is a combination of the word *wanita*, woman, and *pria*, man. Most are transvestites, not transsexuals, and nearly all are sex workers. There are thought to be about 5,000 in Jakarta alone. Their clientele are young Indonesian men and boys, who use the *waria* to experiment with sex. In this Muslim society young men traditionally cannot begin sexual life with women until marriage. The *waria* provide an outlet which serves the dual role of protecting unmarried girls from sexual pressures and allowing young men some sexual release. As in Thailand, the great majority of these young men are 'heterosexual' in orientation, even if their sexual lives begin with transvestite partners.

In one large HIV study done among the *waria*, more than 600 were interviewed and agreed to HIV testing. The average number of sex partners per week was eight; most clients wanted to penetrate the *waria* anally, to have oral sex, or to have 'simulated vaginal intercourse' between the thighs, the intracrural sex favored by the classical Greeks. In 1994, surprisingly, none of these 600 or so transvestites was HIV-infected, despite very high risks (nearly all reported regular receptive anal sex without condoms). HIV rates in their young and sexually inexperienced partners are likely to be low, but the potential for rapid spread is real.

Malaysia also has its transgender community, as does Cambodia, the birthplace of the term *katoey*. India, a root civilization for all the cultures discussed, has her traditional transgender class, though the Indian tradition is something of a special case. There is an excellent discussion of this tradition in the *Kama Sutra*, the Sanskrit classic on sex and sexuality, which describes not only the third gender, but the kinds of intercourse men might have with them (in addition to what must surely be one of the world's earliest treatises on fellatio).

Indian civilization has an awesome ability to see almost anything in terms of the spirit. Prostitution still has a religious gloss in the hereditary temple prostitutes of Rajasthan. Poverty and nakedness, a life of ashes, are the revered garb of the Sadhu. And the Indian 'third gender', the *hinjra*, are called into service by the Divine Mother to serve her cult. There are very few ways permanently to 'lose' caste in India: you can get leprosy, a potent social leveler; you can become enlightened in this lifetime, triumphing over all karma, including a low birth; or you can become a *hinjra*. Unlike in Thailand or Laos, where men who choose (or are born to) this path can stay with their families, in their communities, and live as ordinary women, the Indian *hinjra* becomes an instant outcast, leaving family, community, and caste. She usually joins a band of others like her, and takes up a life of wandering, street performing, begging, and prostitution, if she survives the initiation; many do not.

The initiation into the service of the Goddess is a sacrifice, offered with one swift slice of a knife – penis, scrotum, testicles. Those who survive have typically only a small scarred opening through which to urinate. Infections are common, as are strictures and chronic pain. To serve the Goddess fully, the initiate also plucks (not shaves – too easy!) all of the male body hair. There is one last step in this process: anal dilatation, usually using a wooden dildo set in a special chair, to prepare for a life of selling sex to straight men. (What we do for love!) Thai *katoeys* cross the educational and class spectrum, and are very much aware of HIV and STDs. By 1995, over 40 percent of rural *hinjra* had already acquired HIV.

And the ladies? *Tom* is a Thai word adapted from 'tomboy', an Americanism for a girl with boyish behavior. *Dee*, another Thai expression, is a shortened form of the English 'lady'. *Tom* and *dee* have fairly precise equivalents in English: butch and femme, top and bottom, bulldyke and lipstick lesbian. It is immediately obvious that while words like *katoey* and *hinjra* are ancient, the words used to identify lesbians in Thai culture are very new and very much borrowed from other tongues and topographies. There is an old expression in Thai for sex between women: *lin phuen*, to 'play with friends', but this specifies an act, not a gender or type of woman; both words in this expression are gender-neutral. There may be an unwritten history of lesbian or female transgender traditions in Southeast Asia, but there is very little documentation available. Women's sexuality is (as always) much less discussed, studied, and understood. The traditional 'third genders' are all variations on maleness approaching the female, not the other way around. Seen this way, the *katoey*, the *waria*, the *hinjra* are all forms of Asian male identity: they reflect, perhaps, much more how the societies they come from configure male gender and sexuality, not female. Women, even if men attempt to become them through radical self-mutilation, remain hidden.

One does, however, see the occasional Thai woman in a suit and tie, with a brush cut, speaking the male dialect. If Thai society does not have a name for her, equivalent to *katoey*, she is still fully taking on a male role; such women are not rare, and they seem, in tolerant Thailand at least, socially acceptable. I met one such person in Laos as well, in the entourage of the minister of forestry; we chatted for several minutes in Thai before I realized that the young bureaucrat was a woman. His voice, clothes, and hair were perfect, but you can't fake an Adam's apple.

16 | *CHAAI CHUAY CHAAI*: MEN HELPING MEN

The box arrived one day at my office in Chiang Mai, brimming over with sheets of yellowing paper. It had come from Dr Chawalit's office, from a nurse named Khun Piyada, and it contained the results of five years' work with men working in Chiang Mai's gay bars and clubs. It took some time to sort through the data, get it into shape for analysis, put it together, and understand what it all meant. Buried in these data was epidemiologic gold – a tremendous amount of information on bar-boys and their extraordinary risk of HIV infection, but also evidence that some men had been able to avoid the virus, despite years of selling sex.

Male commercial sex in Thailand is a very different affair from the heterosexual commercial scene. It is a much smaller branch of the industry, localized to essentially five sites: the cities of Bangkok and Chiang Mai, and the beach resorts of Pattaya, Phuket, and Hat Yai. The workers are not trafficked and not, by and large, debtbonded. The sex is considerably more expensive, the pay better for workers. Even in the flesh trade, it's a man's world.

Most male sex workers in northern Thailand were heterosexual outside their work in bars; perhaps 60 percent said they preferred sex with women; about 15 percent were married. This information was in the box from Khun Piyada, and other groups had confirmed similar rates of heterosexual orientation among male sex workers in Bangkok.

Sex work for men in Chiang Mai tended to be much shorter-term than it was for women. The average time in the business was six months, and about one-third of workers did it for two months or less. Women worked an average of two years or more, and debt-bonded women often had to work this long before they began to see any money. Men, in contrast, were selling sex for short-term financial needs, for fast cash. Most were rural men coming to the city for the first time; sex work is a starter's job, and it can pay considerably better than menial labor or restaurant work, other typical first-time employments.

The clients were also a different group. Most Thai men couldn't afford the drinks in a gay bar, much less one of the men. The clients in the gay scene are well-heeled, and the workers reported that about half their clients were not Thai, a much higher percentage than in the heterosexual market. Other Asians were represented, as were Europeans, Australians, North Americans, men from the Middle East. In Hat Yai, on the Thai–Malaysian border, a significant part of the business was Malaysian men. A small minority of clients were women, or heterosexual couples. A small scene has been described on the island of Phuket, where Thai men specialize in providing sex (and entertainment) to Japanese women. Denied casual sex in their own country, a new generation of Japanese women look for it elsewhere.

Thai commercial gay bars are bizarre places, quite unlike what most gay men would recognize as a gay bar in the West: anywhere from ten to forty men hanging around in jock straps, with numbers pinned to their crotches; go-go boys dancing nude, or nearly so; live sex shows; 'captains' circulating, asking if any number strikes your fancy. These are not brothels – the sex happens elsewhere – making the gay bars rough equivalents of 'indirect' or higher-class straight establishments. Customers have to pay the bar to take a worker home; this is the source of the bar's income, along with drinks and cover charges for shows. What the sex worker gets is between him and the customer. Some bars specialize in offering weightlifters or boxer types; others have poetically beautiful young men in tuxedos, or dressed up in traditional Thai formal wear, barefoot and bowing. *Katoeys* are rare in the commercial scene, except as drag-show performers. What clients want is muscular, clean-cut, athletic types – straight farm boys – which is, in fact, mostly what they get.

In the five years' work done by Khun Piyada, we found that, despite the short-term nature of their work, and much higher levels of empowerment and education, male sex workers were nonetheless getting infected with HIV at high, steady rates. These men had, in fact, the highest rates of new HIV infection of any group of men in Asia; from 1989 to 1995 a regular 12 percent per year were getting HIV. This was in addition to the 20 percent of men who were already positive on any cross-sectional look, making gay-bar work about as deadly an occupation as one can imagine. This was hard to reconcile with what seemed to be much better working conditions than those found among female sex workers. These were Thai men, not tribal boys; many were literate; some were university students making pocket money while they studied. Two other findings helped to clarify the situation. Men who had worked longer in the business should have had higher rates, since they would have had many more opportunities for infection. They did not; their rates were lower, and fell progressively over time. This suggested that if men had time to learn about safer sex, they did better at staying uninfected. The second finding was more straightforward: men who said they 'sometimes', 'most often', or 'almost always' used condoms had the same high rate as men who said they 'rarely' or 'never' used them. Only men who said they 'always' used condoms for anal sex were protected. Not a surprise. What was surprising was that condom use was not universal; it was lower than among men in the Thai Army: only 56 percent of male sex workers said they 'always' used condoms. Even in the cheapest brothels, female sex workers were doing better. During the five years of the study, the nurses from the ministry had been giving out free condoms to all the workers, the bars all had them prominently displayed, sex workers asked to show condoms nearly always had some on hand. What was wrong?

The problem was, and is, a complex one, and it is far from solved in 2016. The Ministry of Health program was only able to visit each bar twice a year, so many short-term workers missed it entirely. The data suggested that men new to the business were the least skilled at using condoms, and at avoiding HIV. Sexual orientation did not seem to matter. Men who said they were 'men', 'gay kings', 'gay queens', or '*katoey*' all had roughly the same risk. The crucial time for HIV risk appeared to be the learning phase of sex work, the first few weeks or months on the job, before workers knew how to insist on condom use, and before they themselves were skilled in safe anal sex practices. Most reported that foreign clients were easier to negotiate condom use with than their own countrymen. Thai clients more often demanded anal intercourse and did not want to wear condoms. How to intervene?

With several friends, we developed the concept of a sex workers' group, which would train men working in the industry to be peer educators.[1] This network would identify any new workers in the bars, and get to them with frank practical advice on avoiding HIV before they became infected. We called the group *Chaai Chuay*

Chaai – men helping men. (To 'help', *chuay*, is a Thai euphemism for masturbation, so the name has a second meaning, immediately clear to Thais.) The group got funding from the Australian government, and we were in business. We had five volunteers, all sex workers or ex-sex workers, who regularly visited all the gay bars that would have them, the cruising areas, and the street hustler scenes of nighttown Chiang Mai – places they had all worked and knew intimately. They came back from their shifts with some incredible tales to tell.

One bar did have some non-Thai workers. These were Shan and Burmese who had been brought to Thailand on construction crews. When their road work or construction jobs ended, some of the younger and more handsome ones had been recruited into sex work. Several workers turned out to be Burmese soldiers who had defected from the army, snuck into Thailand, and ended up in the bars as illegal aliens. There were boys from Laos. There was much more drug abuse than the boys had reported to the visiting nurse teams; glue- and thinner-sniffing was common, as was ecstasy, amphetamines, and heavy alcohol use. And there *were* some real brothels. These were very clandestine, strictly Thai establishments without the usual bars or restaurant businesses as covers. Three were found. These places were all private homes, open in the afternoon, when the workers got out of school. Local men came for cheap sex with schoolboys, virtually all of whom were supporting drug habits by selling sex. Reaching them was dangerous, and had to be done with caution. There was also a small pedophile scene, operating out of several bars, where men could arrange for sex with boys as young as eight or nine. As soon as the volunteers reached these places, the children promptly disappeared; these kids proved almost impossible to track down. We started working with a local group that tried to offer housing and support to homeless street kids, and found that many had been part of this pedophile scene; more than half had HIV infection in 1995.

Our volunteers were giving out a lot of condoms and lubricants, and counseling all over the city, night after night. After a year, we eagerly awaited the results from the ministry survey of the bars. Were we having an effect? No, we weren't. HIV rates were steady, despite continuing efforts on the part of the ministry, despite *Chaai Chuay Chaai*, despite the national education campaign which seemed to be working with so many other groups. Gay commercial sex was not getting any safer, and that was where the situation stood in the late 1990s.

Over the next decades a number of things changed for men who have sex with men in Thailand, and for the male sex work industry. In Chiang Mai the workers became less and less Thai and more Shan – as awareness grew among the Thais of the danger of the work. The 2003–2005 law and order campaign of PM Thaksin made the whole scene much less safe as condoms were seen as evidence of promoting homosexuality, and they vanished from the bars and clubs. But the HIV risks, and the very high rates of new infection among these young men didn't change. Didn't budge in fact.

In 2014 we started a new collaboration with SWING, the sex workers union, the U.S. CDC, and the Thai Ministry of Health to assess if PrEP could make a difference for these young men. PrEP has some real potential advantages for young men selling sex. It is highly effective, including for the receptive partner, the bottom, in anal sex. It's under the individual's control, so doesn't require agreement from a client or a lover. It's not cheap enough yet, costing about U.S.$25 per month – and the Thai government is not paying for it through the national health scheme, so most men will have to pay out of pocket. Men in our project who choose to take it will get it free of charge. We should know by 2019 if PrEP finally will break the back of this decades long epidemic. Watch this space.

Several other countries in the region have male commercial sex scenes in addition to Thailand: Sri Lanka and the Philippines are the most commonly cited. Indonesia has a local trade in transvestites; Bali is known for a significant sex tourist scene with gay bars and beach boys, and for an international clientele. What makes Thailand somewhat different is that it is easily the most tolerant and open country in Asia for gay men, for commercial sex patrons, but also for gay men who are not interested in commercial sex. For this group, Bangkok is the new Amsterdam, the New York or Paris of the region. When you go out to the non-commercial bars and clubs of gay Bangkok, you meet Singaporeans, Malaysians, Indonesians, Taiwanese, Indians, Koreans, Japanese, Filipinos, Laotians – men reveling in the freedom of big, hot discos, fabulously louche gay saunas, disinterested police.

2016

Gay Asia is changing fast. The current generation is coming out in ever greater numbers. Pride marches are everywhere – and if not as massive are getting as raucous as they do in Sydney or Cape Town. The ways that men find each other and connect – hook up, for money or romance – are changing too. No more the rest rooms and public parks of their grandfathers' generation, or the bars and clubs of their fathers'. Men now make contact through the same social media apps that have transformed gay men's lives in the West. Grindr and Jack'D, and an array of other geospatial apps, are allowing men to find each other all over the region. This is changing sex work – taking out the middle men, and as in so many other transactions, from car rides to places to stay, allowing buyers and sellers to connect directly. More egalitarian? Perhaps. More safe? Perhaps not. In these interactions, there are no bars to enforce condom use. No basket of free condoms on the counter as you head out the door. Anyone with a smartphone and the interest can partake. We are just beginning to understand how this will play out for the HIV epidemics ongoing in Asia. But it is already clear that the future of HIV spread in the region is, like its past, going to involve all too many of these young men.

Owing to drug abuse, there is also a high prevalence of HIV/AIDS in prisons. Prisoners are always afraid to get injections in the jail hospital because of AIDS. When administering injections, the doctors give only half or less than half of the phial to one patient, giving the rest to another patient from the same needle and syringe, this almost guaranteeing that any blood-carried infections will spread. This means that the doctors can get away with using less medicines per patient.

The following are the usual implements used for beating prisoners:

1. Leather-coated pipe
2. Wooden stick
3. Stick made from three interlaced pieces of cane
4. Solid bamboo stick about 3–4 ft in length
5. Hard plastic water pipe.

(*Cries from Insein: A Report on Conditions for Political Prisoners in Burma*, ABSDF, 1996)

On August 2, 1996, a man died in Yangon General Hospital, having been brought there, near death, from Insein Prison in Burma. His name was U Hla Than. He was an elected member of the Burmese parliament, the body which won the 1990 elections but was never allowed to convene. He was 52 years old. Opposition groups immediately claimed that he had been tortured to death, a common enough occurrence in Insein Prison, which Amnesty International has repeatedly cited for its gross violations of human rights and for the use of torture. The then military dictatorship, SLORC, claimed he died of tuberculosis. Aung San Suu Kyi (who had just been put under *de facto* house arrest again) made a public statement in October about the death of her colleague which contrasted with both of these positions. The MP had been tortured, and he had died of tuberculosis, but neither of these facts were sufficient to tell the whole truth. His tuberculosis was a complication of AIDS, Aung San Suu Kyi wanted to stress. His HIV infection was a complication of his imprisonment, and his imprisonment was for the crime of having been democratically elected. He was not known to be a heroin user or to have been involved in homosexual activities while in prison – as an older man and a political prisoner famous among his people, he was somewhat spared from these threats. But like so many prisoners in Burma's jails, he had been offered food (a single hard-boiled egg is standard, according to survivors) in exchange for blood. Blood-collection equipment in Burma's gulag was routinely re-used without sterilization, as documented above in the account of Win Naing Oo, a young man incarcerated for three years in Insein Prison for participating in the 1988 student movement against the junta. In U Hla Than, another Burmese democracy leader was martyred, the instrument being not a 'hard plastic water pipe' or a bullet, but the human immunodeficiency virus.

Condoms are not available to prisoners in the Thai, Burmese, Malaysian, Indian, or, for the most part, U.S. prison systems. A senior Thai prosecutor told me in the late 1990s that almost any sentence longer than three years was considered tantamount to a death sentence in the prison in Chiang Mai, since prisoners held any longer than this were dying 'like flies' of AIDS. It is a terrible irony of the Thai epidemic that a 1988 national amnesty offered to prisoners (owing to an important anniversary) first released an unknown number of HIV-infected men into the country. Needle sharing and unprotected homosexual sex had spread HIV extensively among these men. Within months of their release, the Thai epidemic was under way.

HIV prevention in prisons has been an abysmal, even criminal failure worldwide. In Asia it has been no better handled than in most prison systems. What made the Burmese and Thai situations so lethal is that HIV rates were already high enough among young men, such that prison acts as an accelerator. Indeed, among addicts in Thailand, having been incarcerated is the single most important difference between men who have HIV and those who do not. HIV infection in Thai addicts is highly correlated with having been jailed. The U.S., to its lasting shame as a nation born to embody freedom, has the highest incarceration rate in the world at about 707 persons per 100,000 population, about 50% higher than in the Russian Federation and more than five times higher than China. South Africa used to be a close second, but has since dropped out of the running, leaving us essentially alone among developed nations in our fervor to imprison our citizens. As befits the new era of privatization, prisons are now profit-making enterprises, with privately operated prisons picking up the slack of the overwhelmed public system. In a stunning ironic twist worthy of Gogol, prisons now mean jobs. One phrase (is it actually true?) has been repeated till it has lost the power to shock: 'There are more young black men in prison than in college in America today.' This has had major impacts on HIV across black communities. It has not been due to HIV transmission in prisons, which occurs but is uncommon, but rather to something more complex. U.S. state and federal prisons actually do a reasonable job of treating incarcerated persons with HIV infection. Jails are less successful. But what is critical is about 14 percent of all Americans living with HIV cycle through the criminal justice system each year. And of course, mass incarceration is primarily a reality for men of color in the U.S. The biggest problem is not infection while in prison, or lack of treatment, but treatment interruptions upon release. When a man or a woman who has been on antivirals abruptly stops, the virus comes roaring back, usually in a matter of a few weeks. It can come back at very high levels, rendering the untreated person highly infectious for sex partners. If both repeated cycles of incarceration and HIV are concentrated in the same community, as they are among black Americans, this becomes a vicious cycle which accelerates HIV spread.

It is hard otherwise to explain the extraordinarily uneven burden of HIV infection among African American women. They have lower individual risks then other American women, yet more than 90 percent of all HIV infections among women in the U.S. are in this relatively small population. The repeated arrest, detention, and treatment interruptions among black men with HIV have acted as a terrible catalyst for HIV in black women.

It is past time to end the war on drugs. And it is past time to use incarceration to address substance use, or to imprison people for being who they are, gay, trans, or a sex worker. Mass incarceration is cruel, inhuman, expensive, and helping to keep the HIV virus alive and well in our human family.

18 | ACTIVISTS

> Humanity's innate desire is for freedom, truth, and
> democracy. The nonviolent 'people power' movements that
> have arisen in various parts of the world in recent years have
> indisputably shown that human beings can neither tolerate
> nor function properly under tyrannical conditions. (Tenzin
> Gyatso, His Holiness the Fourteenth Dalai Lama of Tibet)

Demands for prevention rarely get protestors out on the streets.
Vaccines have had few vocal advocates since the polio scares of
the 1930s and 1940s, except those demanding compensation for
putatively vaccine-related damage to their children. Demands for
care, for access to treatment, have created mass movements, for no
disease perhaps more spectacularly than for AIDS. AIDS activism
brought about changes in the price of drugs (AZT, after activists
chained themselves to the doors of the New York Stock Exchange,
delaying the opening of the world's largest financial market), altered
the way the U.S. Food and Drug Administration approves new agents
(after a series of actions there), and forced the Centers for Disease
Control to review the very definition of the disease (after ACT-UP
occupied the roof of their Atlanta office building). While not all the
outcomes of AIDS activism have been beneficial to people with the
disease, or to researchers, the cumulative effect of public pressure
can be seen in the astonishingly wide array of new treatments now
available, in the anti-viral combination therapies, and in the huge
research investments that have tested their clinical efficacy. We now
have the technology (quantitative viral load testing) to measure viral
responsiveness to these drugs in patients taking them, allowing for
rational and informed decisions about when to change agents, when
to stop them altogether, when to initiate them in a person seemingly
well but in whom the virus has begun aggressive replication. In the
magical years of 1996–1997 I saw friends who were at death's door
begin to gain weight, grow back their hair, get off disability, and go

back to work within three to six months after starting on the new three-drug regimes. This kind of progress would not have occurred without the immense resources appropriated to the NIH (specifically NIAID) under the first Bush and Clinton administrations. But those resources might never have been mustered had it not been for the committed and effective activists on the front lines of confrontation. Who will ever forget ACT-UP's infiltration of the evening news in New York, at the height of the Gulf War, shouting 'Fight AIDS, not Arabs' to a stunned anchorman?

Advocacy for prevention has been another matter.

Thailand has had one activist, Khun Meechai Viravaidya, a prominent citizen who made condom promotion a personal crusade. Khun Meechai used a promotion tactic all too often ignored by Western activists: humor. He appealed to the Thai sense of *sanuk* – fun – using condom flowers, giving condom bouquets to ladies, spreading a message that stressed the 'sex-positive', and the maintenance of pleasure that safer sex could mean in the era of AIDS. Wherever and whenever he appeared, at society balls or at public schools, he gave out condoms. He started a chain of restaurants, called 'Cabbages and Condoms', where all diners received condoms with their meals. So associated did he become with condom use that the slang word for condom in central Thai became 'a *meechai*', and using a *meechai* became synonymous with practicing safer sex. As a member of the Thai elite, Khun Meechai had considerable access to the media and to Thai decision makers, access that he used to promote condoms tirelessly, but always with wit, humor, and appeals to the Thai sense of tolerance and sexual pleasure. While direct effects are always difficult to measure, there is no question that his early and energetic efforts contributed to the rapid nationwide increase in condom use that makes Thailand unique, at least for now, in Asia. In a promising sign that his message may have a regional impact as well, Khun Meechai received Asia's highest humanitarian award, the Magsaysay Prize, in 1995.

Northern Thailand in the late 1990s had more than 60 self-help groups for people with HIV/AIDS. Most came together seeking treatments, including the largest, Pheun Cheewit, New Life Friends, which had over 5,000 members in the Chiang Mai valley. New Life Friends was actually an unwitting creation of the Thai Ministry of Health. In 1994, a herbalist in northern Thailand was making a name selling a herbal remedy for HIV which, he claimed, could make people go from being HIV-positive to HIV-negative. People flocked to him. The great majority, of course, were getting no other treatment, and were never going to afford AZT, the only AIDS drug then available in Thailand. The Ministry was rightly concerned that the man was a profiteer, exploiting people with AIDS for money, of which he was reportedly making plenty. The herbalist was shut down, causing instant uproar among the hundreds of people to whom he had offered, if nothing else, hope. Galvanized, they formed New Life Friends to lobby the government for access to the banned herbal treatment. In classic Thai fashion, a deal was struck: New Life Friends would be recognized as a 'club', members would pay a small monthly fee of 50 Baht (about U.S.$2, well within most Thai pocketbooks) and would then have access to the herbal therapy, which would be free to club members. The club quickly caught on, and later served not only as a mechanism for access to care, but as a social group, a community center, and a place to look for work.

Two other strands of activism emerged early in the Thai epidemic, from two very different groups in society: sex workers and their advocates; and the *sangha*, the monastic community.

Early on in the Thai epidemic there was tremendous fear of people with AIDS. Fear of contagion born of misunderstandings that were only natural given the lack of general awareness at the community level, the newness of the disease, and its high lethality. Finding places to get care was a real problem; many clinics and hospitals turned the early cases away. Finding places to live, and then to die, became even more problematic. The long-term solution was clearly going to have to be home care; this the authorities recognized and promoted, as did the very active Thai Red Cross, which soon began support programs, and has now trained thousands of home-care givers. But in the short term there was a real crisis: people with AIDS were living in parks, isolated like lepers at the outskirts of villages, abandoned by families to the street. The Thai *wat*, the Buddhist temple, has always been a place of refuge. Children without care-givers have long been 'given' to *wats*; widows and childless elderly are often found staying at them, as are young people between jobs, even criminals hiding from the law, or AWOL soldiers. The first Thai *wat* to offer refuge, and to create an AIDS hospice for the dying, was in Lopburi, in the lower north. The abbot, a progressive and powerful figure in Thai monasticism, faced considerable criticism for opening his center. (He had been inspired to do so after a visit to the Shanti Project, the San Francisco AIDS hospice which grew out of a gay men's spiritual circle in the 1980s.) After several years of successful work and growth, it is now the largest such hospice in Thailand, and a focus for donations from the concerned middle and upper classes of the area. It is a beautiful facility, and it offers people in need of pastoral and physical solace a peaceful and meditative refuge. Hundreds of Thais have died there, and hundreds more lived there in the next decades..

In Chiang Mai, things were not as easy for Phra Pongthep, the activist monk who began the city's first AIDS refuge. Phra Pongthep was an unusual man by any measure. He was outspoken and direct, openly critical in a manner many Thais find unnerving. He pushed. When he first conceived of the idea of starting a hospice, the Abbot of his *wat* was strongly opposed. Phra Pongthep simply moved out, to what was essentially a shed near the main *wat*, and began. At first, patients slept in the open air, cared for only by Phra Pongthep and a few volunteers. He persisted, gradually building up the facility through donations. Kai Kawila Army Hospital donated beds and bedding. The Australian government offered money for food and drugs. A taxi driver with HIV infection offered himself and his car to serve as a makeshift ambulance. Still-well people with HIV volunteered to help with the sick. A Dutch nurse spent several months training these volunteers. The place in 1997 looked more like a barn than a hospice, and it was nothing if not simple. It was always filled to capacity and over. Phra Pongthep, however, was not interested in expansion. He firmly believed that people with AIDS, as with any other illness, should be cared for at home. He was blunt with family members seeking to 'drop off' a sick relative. The people at his center were those without families, with nowhere else to go. If a family was at all able, Phra Pongthep worked with them to care for their ill member, and offered the blessing and support which Thais find in their monks. Though a small and slender man, and young by Thai standards for a monk on his own (he is 35), he was a formidable figure, and compelled his listeners with a sharp tongue and quick wit. He was also something of a radical, for many of the people dying at his small center were women, and he had, on occasion, to touch them (when lifting, for example, or checking the progress of a wound). Thai Buddhist tradition is notably conservative on this point: women and monks never have even the slightest physical contact. Women must stand on two legs, never one, in the presence of monks. A woman's laundry may not touch a monk. Phra Pongthep was challenged on the unorthodox nature of his work, and gave this answer:[1]

> Let me tell you a story. Soon after the passing of the Buddha, one of his disciples was walking toward Benares with a young novice. The two monks came to the River Jamuna, which was high after the rains. There was no boat, and they would have to walk across, using sticks. On the shore they found a young woman, stranded, who was too weak to make her way across. The novice was shocked when his old master picked up the woman, put her on his back, and carried her across to the far shore. Once across, the master put her down, and the two monks went on their way. The master said nothing about the event, but the novice was deeply disturbed. That night, he challenged the master: 'How could you have done such a thing?' To which the master replied, 'I only carried her across the river. You have carried her all the way here.'

The other strand of AIDS activism in Thailand, and one which is very much at the center of HIV/AIDS work in Cambodia, has grown out of women's movements in both countries, out of those groups concerned with the rights of women in the sex industry. When HIV hit Thailand, the only organizations already active with women in the sex trade were groups like EMPOWER, an NGO begun by Thai women to assist sex workers in Bangkok, and the Women's Relief Center, a safe-house for battered women run by a Thai Buddhist nun, Mae Chi Khunying Khanitta. The same held true for the Cambodian Women's Development Association, which began as a women's rights body, took up the plight of trafficked sex workers, and is now one of the leading indigenous groups working on HIV prevention and care. These are all service organizations, whose mandates have had to change as HIV overwhelmed the women they were working with.

EMPOWER has the strengths and limitations inherent in the eclectic world of NGOs. It is small, with two offices: one in Bangkok and one in Chiang Mai. Its operating budget is correspondingly small. The group relies heavily on volunteers, and on larger donor agencies for providing the salaries of paid staff. The great strength of an organization like EMPOWER is not its scale, but its grassroots base – the women they work with know them intimately, trust them, share their lives with them. Jackie Pollock, an English teacher, had been with EMPOWER for over a decade, and helped found the Chiang Mai branch. Walking into a local brothel with Jackie was a lesson in the kind of relationships such commitment can build. If you stepped in as a man alone you'd see women and girls sitting around like rabbits: blank stares, little talk, faces flat and vague. When these same women saw Khun Jackie they'd burst into life, instantly becoming themselves – village girls again, full of warmth, hugging and laughing and talking. They loved her, and in the loveless life of a sex worker, such human connections may be one of the few ties to hope.

EMPOWER began working with women in the sex trade well before HIV spread in Thailand. By 1996, about half the women they worked with had HIV, and many were beginning to progress to AIDS, to die. What began as a service organization committed to empowering sex workers had to cope with getting women (often illegal residents – about half are from Burma) medical care, and safe places to convalesce, and to pass. It is a sad reality of Thai medicine that sex workers generally get very poor care. They are rarely treated with respect, if they get any treatment at all. Once HIV-infected, they get even less, their treatable symptoms dismissed as 'just a part of AIDS'. With an EMPOWER nurse along for their clinic visits or hospitalizations, they at least had an advocate. In the Thai context this was invaluable. Even the poorest of the poor are treated differently if they have a patron. If the patron is a foreigner, all the better.

Social activism of this kind is tolerated only with the strictest of government controls in the three communist states of the region, China, Laos, and Vietnam. Advocates for social or political change in these countries are routinely jailed, put in labor camps, or they disappear. China's treatment of AIDS activists is well known – many have had to flee the country. Vietnam, despite its recent 'opening' to capitalist markets, is not much better; the Vietnamese regime continues to hold in prison senior Buddhist monks and Catholic priests who have resisted Communist Party control of their institutions. The 75-year-old abbot of one of the country's principal Buddhist monasteries had his imprisonment extended another four years (to a total of eight) in 1996. His crime? Having assisted flood victims without permission from the Party. When I asked one of his disciples why he thought this 'crime' was being punished so harshly, he had this to say:

> It is a question of ideology. The Party in power here believes in Marxist-Leninist-Maoist ideology. They cannot accept that Buddhism sees man differently. They are afraid of the peoples' love for our teacher here, and so they jail him. Actually, this is very irrational. If you take what people want away, try to destroy it, they will want it more. But our problem now is that our teacher is a very old man, and he is not well. They have denied us any real teaching here, and he is taken from us. So our Buddhist traditions are not being preserved and transmitted. I believe this regime will change, but by then it may be too late.

The price of social activism in Southeast Asia is high. In Burma, from 1962 until 2011, those Burmese who challenged the successive military regimes risked harassment, exile, prison, torture, extra-judicial execution, and the persecution of their families and contacts. That so many people have been willing to pay this price for so long is a testament to how deep the yearning for justice can be, how compelling the thirst for freedom. While superficially more law-abiding and progressive countries such as Thailand and Malaysia would seem to be safer for dissenters, both have exiled, jailed, and killed social activists with impunity. Seven people were assassinated in the build-up to Thailand's 1996 national elections. Labor and environmental leaders have been murdered, including the activist leader of The Forum for the Poor, a farmers' lobby that was trying to prevent a dam project from forcing the relocation of farming families in Thailand's impoverished northeast. In 1995 a community hospice for people with AIDS was fire-bombed in Thailand. Malaysia has jailed most of the leaders of a conservative Muslim political movement there. AIDS activism in Southeast Asia has thus far not pushed for political reform; its focus has been on relatively less threatening calls for an end to discrimination, access to care, and dignity in death. Given the current political climate for dissent, AIDS activists in Asia are likely to face regimes sorely tested by their demands. AIDS activism may challenge and invigorate Buddhist movements as well. His Holiness the Dalai Lama of Tibet has called on the Buddhist clergy to become more engaged in worldly problems, citing the Christian clergy's involvement with liberation theology as an example of what Buddhism must do to stay relevant and alive. Maha Ghosananda echoed this call for the Cambodian clergy. Nowhere has it been more strongly taken to heart than in Burma, where monks and nuns marched for democracy in their hundreds of thousands, in the Saffron Revolution. How many committed monks and nuns like Phra Pongthep are there still in the prisons of Vietnam and China?

PART THREE

RELATIVITY AND CULTURE

Why have we not responded? Working at one of the nation's finest academic institutions, I have sought advice from faculty colleagues in American history, law, and public health as to why our national response to the AIDS epidemic has been so inadequate. I have tried to find out what it is about our past that makes it so difficult for us to deal rationally with an epidemic of a fatal sexually transmitted disease. Two things are apparent. First, as a nation we have never 'conquered the Victorian within ourselves', preferring to deny our sexual behavior even when the behavior presents an untold risk to ourselves and our loved ones. Second, because HIV infection is contagious and presumed fatal, and AIDS is a disfiguring illness at its end stage that elicits fears about our own mortality, we have stigmatized AIDS and those populations with high rates of HIV infection. It is especially unfortunate that many of those infected have been from populations already stigmatized because of sexual orientation, race, occupation (e.g. sex workers), or other behavior (e.g. injecting drug use). (Michael H. Merson, 'Returning home: reflections on the USA's response to the HIV/AIDS epidemic', *The Lancet*, 1996)

19 | DRUG WARS AND THE WAR ON DRUGS

War and the social chaos and upheavals it brings make an almost ideal setting for epidemic diseases (from the Greek *epi demos*, 'upon the people'). There are no more moving descriptions of the toll these diseases exact than Walt Whitman's. The poet served as a field nurse in several military hospitals during the American Civil War and later published his war remembrances in *Specimen Days*, an unjustly neglected classic of his prose. Whitman watched young man after young man die of typhoid, burn out with fevers, waste away from diarrhea, and endure the miserable end of gangrene and repeated amputations – diseases for which treatment was almost non-existent at the time. The losses were immense, and because it was a civil war, all were ours. Among the soldiers, but particularly among women and children, malnutrition compounded the threat of epidemic diseases. Combine these threats, and war always does combine them, and it becomes clear that more people, and usually more civilians, lose their lives to breakdowns in food distribution, sanitation, and basic health care than to bullets, bombs, or executions. This appears to have been the case during the Khmer Rouge period: while 500,000 people are thought to have been murdered, another 1.5 million Cambodians are thought to have died of malnutrition, disease, and exhaustion from overwork.

For the modern West, epidemics of cholera or typhus, of death from gangrene and staph infections, are a part of distant memory, horrors of historical interest. But most 'modern' wars (and it need hardly be said that the scores of conflicts raging or simmering today are largely civil wars) are fought in field conditions no better than those of nineteenth-century America. You don't find antibiotics for typhoid fever in South Sudan, or disposable surgical equipment in the jungles of Burma; soldiers lose legs, and civilians die, in the same squalor and pain as they did on the battlefields of the American Civil War. Health conditions in the Rwandan conflict were more like Old Testament-era pestilence and made 1860s Virginia look modern. The Hutu prisoners accused of genocide, an estimated 90,000 persons,

were housed in prisons so crowded and filthy that many lost feet
and legs from standing in pooled human feces and urine several feet
deep. For the people of Somalia, DR Congo, Aleppo, the Rohingya
at sea in the Bay of Bengal, modern medical advances might as well
have happened on the moon.

An early slogan of AIDS prevention campaigns in the U.S. was
'AIDS does not discriminate'. While a useful battle cry, this is
unfortunately only partly true. AIDS does discriminate: HIV spreads
fastest where social life is chaotic, where poverty is endemic, where
women are uneducated, and where the rights of vulnerable groups
and individuals are violated. This is true in the world's poorest and
most strife-torn nations, and it is true among the poor of rich nations,
such as the U.S., where HIV spread continues to be localized in
pockets of poverty and social disruption, the red states of the deep
South, where health care access is still denied citizens on the basis of
poverty and social exclusion. Civil war is perhaps the extreme case
of social disruption; human rights violations are part and parcel of
these conflicts, and so it may be only logical that HIV/AIDS should
discriminate against peoples caught in the throes of civil strife. This
may sound an uncommon interaction, but civil war and its social
and health consequences are anything but uncommon in our time.
HIV is only one of many infections that spread rapidly when social
orders are chaotic, blood is being spilled, and women raped. But
unlike cholera, which so devastated the Rwandan refugees, or
malaria, which decimates the freedom fighters of Burma, HIV,
with its stealthy incubation and trivial first symptoms, does not fit
the usual mode of war-related disease outbreaks. To use a military
analogy, cholera goes off like a cluster bomb; HIV seeds a country
like landmines, an analogy of painful aptitude for Cambodia. This is
not a given of course, HIV has to be circulating in a population for
conflict or disruption to drive it – but when both are present, lasting
consequences can result.

Aside from the direct impact of civilian casualties in war (including
landmines), the social disruption of civil unrest can be fertile ground
for more complex health effects. The list of countries where spread
of HIV has been facilitated by political repression, social disruption,
and civil strife is long, and includes at least Uganda in the 1970s
and 1980s, Zaire, Kenya, Rwanda, Burundi, and Haiti. Could the
argument be turned around as well? Could the loss to AIDS of heads

of households, wage earners, the educated and traveling adults of these countries be a component cause of social disruption, of chaos? This is perhaps an impossible question to answer. But these losses, and the burdens they have placed on societies, could plague places like northern and eastern Burma, the Shan and Kachin hills, if and when they finally find peace.

A twist of the civil conflict now threatening Burma's transition to democracy is that it is intimately connected to the heroin and methamphetamine trades. It has been labeled a 'drug war', with all the negative implications such a label carries. This was also the case in Afghanistan in the *Mujahedeen* period and Colombia during her civil war, where drugs bought munitions, and where the porous borders and lawlessness of longstanding conflict made narcotics trafficking comparatively easy. War is good for the drug business, the return of civil society and the rule of law a problem. The black-market cash-flows that drugs generate enrich and empower just those anti-democratic and violent elements who then have a stake in seeing civil conflicts continue. This forces insurgents into a Faustian bargain: they need guns, and may have to allow narcotics production to get them, but this very process undermines their aims, if these should be, as in the case of the Shans and Wa, the defeat of an oppressive (Burman) military presence and a return to civilian rule. Once a conflict is labeled a 'drug war', the international community shuns it; the media often pull out as well, all other elements of the struggle are subsumed under the rubric of 'narcoterrorism' or 'drug warlordism'. This has been the enduring tragedy of the Shan people: since their leaders have been implicated in heroin production, their aspirations have been trivialized. Civilians in this conflict get little support in the UN or from relief agencies.

The heroin trade starts, of course, with farmers.[1] In the case of the Shan, Wa, Kachin, and Hmong, these are subsistence farmers, peasants and civilians. Of the immense revenues their opium crops generate, they see only pennies. The farmers of these hidden hills might do better for their families growing coffee or tea, grain or cotton. But the men with the guns, from both rebel and national armies, want them – in some areas force them – to grow poppies. Billions of dollars a year come out of these hills, and the ordinary people are in rags. Those with energy and courage try to escape, to find work in Thailand, where much of the profit is laundered, invested, and goes on to generate more wealth. But not for them; they just build the buildings.

The Swedish researcher and author Bertil Lintner, and his wife, a Shan social activist, are undoubtedly the leading experts on the complex narcotics industry in Burma, on its political roots and implications. In his encyclopedic study *Burma in Revolt: Opium and Insurgency since 1948*, Lintner argues convincingly that the narcotics trade in Burma cannot be understood outside the context of the civil war, and that only a political solution in the Shan and Wa states can possibly lead to a reduction in opium dependency. He stresses that the narcotics control agencies in the West active in Burma (including the U.S. Drug Enforcement Agency, the DEA) have focused almost entirely on criminalizing the trade, seeing it somehow as an aberration, and not as an intrinsic component of both the insurgents and the military. The logical outcome of the DEA approach would be to offer assistance to Burma's narcotics control program, which the U.S. has done in the past. The problem with this, Lintner argues, is that the military, or people within it, are also involved. Strengthening them may do no more than increase their market share of the heroin trade, and empower them in the struggle against the Shans. Whatever we may think about this argument, recent events in Burma would suggest that Lintner is correct in his assertion. The most powerful leader in the Shan states for much of the 1980s and 1990s was a man named Khun Sa, also known as Chang Chifu, a Chinese-Shan warlord. His Mong Tai Army (MTA) once had 15,000 well-armed fighters, and controlled a significant portion of the Shan states. His insurgency was widely known to be supported on Shan opium, though he also controlled several lucrative jade mines. Khun Sa was labeled U.S. enemy number one by the DEA. House leaders like Representative Charlie Rangel of New York, concerned about the devastation heroin was bringing to his district (Harlem), asked for lethal aid for the DEA and SLORC to capture Khun Sa and bring him to justice. But in early 1996, in a surprise move that threw the Shan states (and U.S. policy) into disarray, Khun Sa 'surrendered' to the SLORC. The U.S. State Department immediately called for his extradition to stand trial for narcotics trafficking, and publicly offered SLORC a U.S.$2 million ransom for him. SLORC refused (U.S.$2 million, considering that Khun Sa reportedly ran as much as one-third of the world's heroin business, is an almost laughable sum – we are talking here about wealth on another scale). Instead, the *New Light of Myanmar*, SLORC's mouthpiece, began referring to Khun Sa as U Khun Sa, signifying a respected elder. SLORC and U Khun Sa later embarked on a joint-venture bus company.

There were no winners in this tango, but many losers. The DEA lost credibility throughout the region, as it was once again confirmed that they 'don't get it'. Harlem lost. But no one suffered more than the Shans. Many supported Khun Sa because of his populist, Shan nationalist rhetoric. He was supposed to be fighting SLORC, and leading the Shans toward independence, or at least autonomy within a federal union. He sold his people to SLORC without their permission and without warning. Two factions split from the MTA over the surrender, led by commanders who wanted to keep the Shan resistance alive. SLORC, however, quickly overran the Shan states. Three-way fighting soon broke out between the SLORC, the Wa, and the Lahu in the Shan states – a land grab/drug war/criminal enterprise that further ravaged the Shans. The farmers of the hills are still growing opium at gunpoint two decades later.

Spill-overs of the Burma–Laos heroin trade, and increasingly, the methamphetamine trade, have continued to cause problems for other countries in the region, notably India and China. The road leading out of the western Chin hills and into India's frontier state of Manipur long carried opium out by the truckload. Manipur, closed to the world through years of ethnic insurgency, now has one of India's worst heroin addiction problems, and among the highest HIV rates of any state in the country. Indian Nagaland, just to the north of Manipur and also a transshipment for heroin out of Myanmar, now has the highest HIV prevalence in all of India. Ethnic peoples on both sides of this border are heavily affected, and heroin is reaching India's cities and her youth. The Burmese spill-over into China, as discussed in the section on China, amounted to perhaps 80 percent of China's entire HIV burden in 1996, making control of Burma's heroin trade an issue of national importance for China as well as for India. But China's position remains murky.

China wants the hydroelectric power, the water itself, of Burma's great central river, the Irrawaddy, which has its origins, like the other great rivers of Asia, in Tibet. The Irrawaddy flows from Tibet, through parts of what is now Yunnan, and into the Kachin State of Myanmar, where the conflict rages. The Burmese military was accused of shelling civilians in camps in Kachin in October 2016. Timber, jade, and drugs continue to flow north from Kachin into China. For now, the vast Irrawaddy continues to flow south, and the plans for China's massive dam, the Myitsone, are on hold. The forests surrounding the great river in Kachin State, however, are already gone. This was supposed to be the largest preserve for the endangered tigers of Asia. It has been clear cut to feed China's insatiable demand for hardwood. When I asked a friend, a Kachin environmental activist, about the preserve, she said, 'I hope the tigers can learn to eat sugar cane. That is all that is growing there now'.

The region's heroin and methamphetamine cartels are reported to be largely controlled by ethnic Chinese clans. These, historically, were outgrowths of the Chinese Nationalist forces (Kuomintang – KMT) that remained trapped in Yunnan and Burma when Chiang Kai Shek fled to Taiwan after his defeat by Mao and the Communists. Old links and clan ties have remained, and seemingly outlasted ideological conflicts. The opium grown in Burma and Laos, and refined in Laos, moves via Kunming to Shanghai, Hong Kong, and then to the West, where it is sold. The picture emerges of a new opium war, but one inverted from the nineteenth-century opium war which so devastated China. In the earlier conflict, India was the farmland for opium; the British were the cartel, carrying opium to China's ports. Britain made an immense fortune from the revenue, which was invested in London. China was humiliated, weakened, and impoverished. Now the cartels are Chinese, the markets in the West, and the cities rising to new heights on the revenues are Shanghai and Kunming. Poetic justice, perhaps, but in both opium wars the casualties are high, the money stained with blood.

The War on Drugs, as opposed to these drug wars, has given us another set of problems. First and foremost, the U.S. has failed to fulfill its end of the bargain – reducing demand. Heroin in 2016 is more plentiful, cheaper, and more powerful than at any time in the past. It has replaced cocaine in many settings as the major hard drug of abuse. Coming on the heels of an epidemic of synthetic and prescription opioid use and abuse, with drugs like oxycontin and codeine, heroin is now being used across the U.S. The affected regions include new zones like New England and Appalachia where overdose deaths have become a major killer of young adults.

The U.S. War on Drugs has been an expensive policy failure. We have jailed hundreds of thousands of Americans to no avail and to lasting harm to individuals, families, and communities. Drug treatment lags in research, in access, and in scope. And, as we've discussed, the HIV preventive measures that could reduce the harm of heroin use, like needle exchanges, have proven difficult to mount in America, which continues to see drug use as criminal behavior, deserving punishment more than treatment. The War on Drugs has been as manifest a failure as our DEA policies in Burma. In both cases, the suffering that has ensued as a result of these failures is immense. Are there other approaches, however politically unfeasible in the current climate of opinion?

Without a political settlement to the Myanmar civil conflict, the country will continue to export heroin and methamphetamine. The military's treatment of U Khun Sa has shown that they cannot be expected to resolve the problem – they are in too deep. ASEAN, India, Europe, Japan, and the U.S. should recognize these realities and use all pressure available, to bring about real negotiations in Myanmar. To bring to the table the military, the National League for Democracy government, and the ethnic nationalities for substantive resolutions of the deadlock. This is what the Shans and Kachins have called for over many decades.

Crop substitution programs, supported by the U.S., have proven quite successful in decreasing opium production in Thailand, now no longer a significant grower. Part of the success of this program, undoubtedly, was the openness and transparency of the Thai state to U.S. officials, researchers, and even tourists, in the hills. With a political resolution in Myanmar and greater openness in Laos, these approaches might succeed again. Significant development funds from donor agencies are also certainly going to be needed to help develop viable alternative economies.

If the current crop were reduced, there would be less heroin in the world market coming from the golden triangle. What effect would that have? Opium growing is already well established in Mexico and Central America, where the cartels have introduced the poppy as a new cash crop. And the regional cartels have already diversified into methamphetamines. If demand remained unchanged, wouldn't the growers simply go elsewhere? Little research is being done on the treatment of opiate addiction. Methadone is an old and imperfect treatment, but one of the few agents in use. We urgently need research into new and better treatment methods, and into drug prevention programs that work. A two-pronged attack of reduced supply (and therefore greater cost) and better treatment might make a real dent in the heroin problems of the U.S. and Europe. Treatment for amphetamine dependency, for other stimulants and synthetics, is even less advanced – there is no methadone equivalent, and no gold standard of behavioral or other therapeutic approaches with compelling evidence of success.

In the meantime, HIV-preventive measures, such as needle exchange, need to be implemented broadly; needle exchange can also help get addicts into treatment, a rare win-win in our losing war on drugs.

How do we get out of this failed war? While the U.S. federal government, even under President Obama, has been largely unable to move past the zero tolerance policies of the past, the states have become innovators. The rapidly changing laws on cannabis, from medical marijuana laws to fully decriminalizing cannabis, including for recreational use, are probably the clearest signs that the zero toler-ance consensus is unraveling. That young people (disproportionally young minority men) are still having their lives upended with can-nabis possession charges in some states, while use is legal in others, is clearly not equal protection under the law. And many states are finding mass incarceration simply too expensive to support.

20 | BRETHREN: HIV, GAY MEN, AND PREVENTION EQUITY

For Clive Van Den Berg

The recognition of the beauty of men, our desire to be with them, dawns early for most gay men. We remember the strange, usually unwelcome feelings. This starts in later childhood for many, by adolescence for most, later for a few who may not grasp their 'difference' until manhood. For most of us these awakenings come with a mix of fear and shame, loneliness and longing. For the fortunate younger generations coming up now, in those fortunate places where LGBTQ people have full civil liberties, for those in accepting families, this is changing. But for most of us, even in 2016, it is still tough to accept who we are, harder to share it with those we love, and most difficult of all to be out and open in public – in schools, on the street, at work. And it need hardly be said that in many places being open about our sexuality, our identities, can lead to social exclusion, violence, even death. While the number has fallen, it is still illegal for consenting adults to engage in same-sex behavior in 73 countries.

There is no legal sanction against homosexuality in Thailand, Cambodia, Laos, Vietnam, or China. The two former British colonies in the region, Burma and Malaysia, share the infamous colonial era 377A penal code criminalizing 'carnal acts against the order of nature'. In the case of Burma, this once included banishment for life, imprisonment, and fines. Malaysia did not have the removal component, but added whipping. The International Lesbian and Gay Association, ILGA, notes that the Malaysian sodomy law has been used almost exclusively against just one person, opposition political leader Anwar Ibrahim, who was sentenced to another five-year term for sodomy in 2015. The law is essentially a dead letter in the Myanmar of 2016 as well, though social sanction against gay people is commonplace.

Southeast Asia has long had peculiar relationships to male sexuality that belie easy categorization of tolerant or intolerant places for gay men. This is perhaps nowhere more the case than in Thailand. Thai women place high value on men's attributes such as softness, politeness, kindness, cleanliness. Men who are courting use the women's dialect to show their tenderness. Visitors to Thailand from the West are sometimes surprised by how openly gay Thais can be – over the seeming tolerance for transgender women, ladyboys, as they are known on the street. But many Thai men struggle mightily with acceptance, with the disappointment they will bring to their families should they come out. Not marry women. Not father. Burma under the generals was a place of an assertive, aggressive masculinity – but the extravagant drag of the *Nat Pwe* mediums persisted. Young Burmese in Yangon at least, are out and happening, with vibrant looks and open affection. Yet no openly gay bars or clubs have been allowed, and Yangon's first gay spa was closed by the authorities soon after opening. As with so many other aspects of Burmese life, the people are way ahead of their leaders. Malaysia, with its British legacy and statist Islam, is an outlier in the region on official tolerance, at least. In 2015 the tourism minister, Datuk Seri Nazri Aziz, stated bluntly that lesbian, gay, bisexual, and transgender Malaysians would never have equal rights. Formerly tolerant Indonesia has recently begun a harsh campaign of anti-gay rhetoric – a surprise to many in the region, and one where some see the impact of conservative (Saudi, Wahhabist) funding and influence at play.

Southeast Asia is changing. Gender norms are changing. But from the perspective of HIV, the single most important change in the past two decades has been the decline in heterosexual transmission and the concomitant increase in HIV burdens among the region's gay and bisexual men. In a global review of the epidemiology of HIV among men who have sex with men, we reported on this phenomenon in 2012, calling these 'dislinked epidemics', since the trajectories were so clearly diverging. We saw this same pattern in the epidemics in South and East Asia, across Western Europe, and in North, Central, and South America and in the Caribbean. In Africa, the continent with the greatest burdens of HIV in heterosexually active women and men, gay African men still had markedly higher rates than straight men. When we pulled all of these data together, and I sat going through the numbers, my heart sank. After all my generation had been through in the 1980s and 1990s, the next generation of gay men was again the community most at risk for HIV. How could this be happening?

Simple explanations are many, and rarely hold. When confronted with the new gay epidemic, easy answers seem at the ready: 'we've forgotten what it was like before treatment'; 'this is because the dying stopped'; 'its chemsex; it's hook up apps and the end of the gay bar culture'; 'its still self-loathing and internalized homophobia driving men toward risk'. All of the above. None of the above.

What does the science say?

We have learned a great deal about HIV transmission and acquisition over the four decades of the pandemic. We now know our early thinking about individuals and their risks as the crux issue was crude and simplistic. What matters is not simply what each of us does or doesn't do with our sexual partners. Gender matters. The colon matters (more on that in a moment), and who we partner with matters. HIV spreads not just between two people, but through chains of transmission in what social scientists call sexual networks. With no other reservoir than each other, this is a virus that requires the most intimate of human contact for spread. But each act of intimacy between two people is nested within a larger context, a web of connectivity, that has huge impact on whether we are likely to acquire HIV or not. A young woman in Norway or Sweden with the typical three or four serial sex partners in her teenage years has essentially no likelihood of acquiring HIV, even if she never sees a condom. A teenage girl of the same age, with the same number of partners as her Swedish sister, but in a black township outside Durban or Cape Town, has a one in five chance of becoming HIV infected by age 21. What's different? The sea in which they are swimming. HIV is vanishingly rare among the heterosexual men in one setting, all too common, and commonly untreated, in the other. The characteristics of the networks we are in shape our risks profoundly, and in ways we rarely perceive. Black gay men in Baltimore have individual risk profiles somewhat more modest than white gay men – they have on average fewer sex partners, somewhat better condom use, and are less likely to mix sex and drugs. HIV rates in 2014? For white men, about 14 percent. For blacks? Try 52 percent, over half. A young black man coming of age in this network and sexually active with men has over a 60 percent lifetime probability of HIV acquisition. This is because the men he is likely to interact with are so likely to have undiagnosed and untreated HIV infection. To have untreated syphilis. And to have neither a physician nor health insurance. Networks matter more than individual behavior.

Biology matters too. (This is where the colon comes in.) Careful analyses of both gay and straight couples who practice anal sex have yielded estimates of the per act and per partner transmission likelihood of anal versus vaginal sex. HIV is transmitted about 18 fold as efficiently across the rectal tissues than across the vaginal ones. That is an enormous difference in probability of infection given an exposure. It is a gut tropic virus, as it turns out, meaning it has a natural propensity for infecting the tissues that line our colons, and that is equally true for men and women – this is not a gay issue but a rectal one. Recent science has also taught us that the first great assault of the virus after infection is the critically important immune system of the gut (called the GALT, for gut-associated lymphoid tissue). After HIV infection, in a matter of weeks, there is about an 85 percent die off of the GALT, and full recovery does not occur even after treatment starts.

There is more bad news. The high transmission probabilities in anal sex are overwhelmingly for the receptive partner – in straight sex only the woman. But gay men can engage in both insertive (top) and receptive (bottom) sex. This means we can engage in the highest risk behavior for acquiring HIV *and* the highest risk behavior for transmitting it. This sex role versatility makes for highly efficient spread within networks of gay men. Role versatility is a gender issue, and one which markedly favors spread between men.

Infectiousness for others is highest during acute and recent HIV infection, before the body's own defenses kick in and get some control of viral replication. No one is more infectious for their sex partners than someone who has just recently become infected – and these people are naturally unlikely to know their status and very unlikely to be treated even if they do. New infections are more common among the young, established (and treated) among older men. The high infectiousness of newly acquired HIV helps drive transmission among young men and allows for especially rapid spread of HIV in their networks. Painful as it is to write this – this is precisely where we are in the fourth decade of AIDS – with higher rates of new infection among young gay men than we have seen in decades.

If there is one consistent finding across the epidemics of HIV in Southeast Asia in 2016 it is the high rate of new infections among young gay and bisexual men.

The future

The new findings from biology, epidemiology, and network science are challenging in that they suggest gay men may long be at great risk for HIV. But they are also liberating. Understanding the high transmission probability across the colon makes HIV prevention much more a biological issue than a moral one. And moving from simplistic incorrect views about individual behavior to more nuanced understanding of why a network and its characteristics might put a young man with only a few partners in life at extraordinarily high risk of acquiring HIV may mean we are willing to judge him less and help him more.

Perhaps most vitally it means we need prevention tools and technologies that are fit to the specific issues relevant for our communities. In the prevention landscape of today, that means we need rapid deployment of two essentials. First, it is critical that gay men already living with the virus get tested and get on treatment. That step, in turn, mandates that gay men can get HIV testing in settings of safety and in dignity, without fear of discrimination or legal sanction. As long as there remain significant numbers of untested and untreated men in our sexual networks, spread will continue. Second, we need to reduce the number of men susceptible to HIV in transmission networks. For now, this means pre-exposure prophylaxis, PrEP, tailored for those who need it most. This is prevention equity. Now that we have the science in hand, not acting on it is indefensible on either medical, public health, or human rights grounds.

PrEP looks to be essential to this equation. One of the reasons PrEP works so well to prevent transmission among gay men is again colonic in nature. PrEP is taken orally, absorbed and concentrated in the lining of the gut. Since gay men's exposure to the virus is also almost entirely through the gut route, this is a potent alignment of risk and protection. It is less clear, for example, how well oral PrEP does in protecting the vaginal compartment from HIV – different route of exposure, different biology – and this may be at least partly why PrEP outcomes in women in risk have been less consistently favorable than the data for men who have sex with men. But for gay men it works remarkably well. Men taking it report experiencing sex without fear of contagion for the first time in decades, or in their lives. They are reporting better, more meaningful relationships, as the discussions around sex, safety, and intimacy are more open and honest with PrEP in the conversation. Risks are not measurably increasing – these are men who met the risk criteria for PrEP by definition – so fears of sharp declines in condom use are not bearing out. Can you hear the hallelujahs from the rooftops? That our time of heightened vulnerability is at last coming to an end?

That the PrEP rollout has been so slow and inconsistent in the midst of this new global epidemic among our young men is a profound frustration. It is also a human rights issue. Taiwan became the first Asian country to make the decision to offer PrEP to her gay men, in October 2016, more than five years after the first successful trial of the drug for prevention. Thailand and Malaysia have both approved use of the medication – but are not willing to pay for it through public systems. China piloted PrEP, rather badly, and looks set to not approve its use despite the severity of her epidemic. It is hard not to see evidence of homophobia in the lack of urgency for implementing a new tool that could control spread among our young people. And indeed, I have heard anti-gay views in conversations, in questions, from health officials in China and Brazil, Thailand, Burma, and the U.S. 'Why should we be paying for these boys to party?' 'Why won't they just use condoms?' 'This is a club drug that encourages unsafe sex.' Again the moralism, the judgment, the sense that our lives matter less. That HIV infection is what we get for our sexual adventuring. This is not what the science is telling us. The best thinking we have now is that young men coming of age and entering networks where HIV is spreading are at high risk for infection given very moderate risks. Some men may indeed use PrEP as a party drug – these are precisely the men we would like to see not become infected and not pass on the virus. And remember, Truvada is a cheap drug in all but the G8 countries, where price supports keep the costs inflated. India and Thailand manufacture it for pennies for their treatment programs.

We can do this. Will we?

To make early treatment and PrEP accessible to those who need them, we're going to need the kind of AIDS activism that played such critical roles in getting AIDS treatments developed and approved in the 1980s and 1990s, and made it available worldwide in the 2000s. For that, we need to stop thinking of this as a pricey prevention option for the well heeled and well informed of Paris and San Francisco and see the right to access PrEP as a fundamental issue to the right to health, to avoiding HIV, to life itself, for people who need and want it. It can be cheap, available, and effective. But we will have to fight.

A human rights case for PrEP can be made on at least two grounds: equity and dignity. Equality is defined (by Webster's) as the state of being equal, of a correspondence in quantity, degree, value. Equity is that which is fair and just. Prevention equity, which I called for in a plenary at South Africa's national AIDS conference in 2015, is fair and just access to HIV prevention technologies for those who need them. Not everyone is at risk for HIV acquisition – indeed, the great majority of humanity is at very low risk if any at all. But young women in South Africa's hard hit communities certainly are. As are young gay men in too many countries. For them, prevention equity means PrEP access.

Dignity is broader. It is the underpinning of the universality of human rights. The state we all share by virtue of being human. Hard to define, but sharply clear to those who have suffered its violations. To have a severe epidemic affecting your community, and to have a tool which works to stop it, and to be denied the chance to protect yourself is a violation of dignity.

Gay men, indeed all sexual and gender minorities, have had few more consistent champions of our fundamental human dignity than His Grace, Archbishop Desmond Tutu of Cape Town. A man with an unfailing moral compass, a beady eye for injustice and huge love for humanity in all its diversity, he has used his global voice to uplift LGBT people early and consistently.

For *The Lancet* special issue we did on HIV among men who have sex with men, I asked the Archbishop (Father, as I am blessed to call him) to contribute a short piece aimed at gay youth. Here is Father:

Why We Have No Choice
Archbishop Emeritus Desmond Tutu

In my beloved country, South Africa, we know all too much about the human cost of prejudice, of discrimination. We learned through painful decades what exclusion can mean, and what terrible and lasting effects it can have for the health and well-being of individuals, families and communities. The apartheid system legalized discrimination based on racial categories. It said, in essence, you blacks are inferior. You deserve less because of who you are and what color you were born. This was a crime against the majority of the people of my country. But it was also a crime against God. For I know in my heart, I know as all faith traditions teach, that there are no inferior people in his eyes. No one deserves less of God's love, less of his mercy, or less of his justice. The papers in this series on HIV among men who have sex with men (MSM) tell us about how far we have to go in providing care, in acceptance, in ceasing to withhold our love. They also tell us what we each already know, if we are prepared to be honest with ourselves – that lesbian, gay, bisexual and transgender people are a part of every human community. LGBT people already have God's full love and acceptance – they are his children too. But they need our acceptance, our love. And to the extent that legal discrimination, those old laws and statutes that make them inferior still exist, it is up to all to work to change those laws. I have no doubt that in the future, the laws which criminalize so many forms of human love and commitment will look the way the apartheid laws do to us now – so obviously wrong. So terribly wasteful of human potential.

Yet I am so heartened in my 80th year by the young people I meet all over the world, who seem to already know this, and have moved so far from intolerance. They are our hope for a more accepting and loving world. And for the LGBT youth out there who are struggling, who are made to feel inferior, let me say this: God loves you as you are. He wants you to live and to thrive. So please take care of yourself, educate yourself about HIV, protect your partners, honor and cherish them. And never let anyone make you feel inferior for being who you are. When you live the life you were meant to live, in freedom and dignity, you put a smile on God's face.

We had a strong series of great scientific papers in this *Lancet* series – on prevention, clinical care for gay men, on the severe epidemic among black men in the U.S., on human rights, on community responses. But what was picked up by the media worldwide, with more than 1,200 stories, what lit up social media, was Father's words about how the current anti-gay laws would look, in the future, as wrong as apartheid looks to us now.

And, of course, they will.

21 | MEDICAL ETHICS, HUMAN RIGHTS, ASIAN VALUES

> AIDS-related human rights activism, sharing the orientation
> of mainstream human rights, has focused on the visible and
> purposeful governmental acts that jeopardize individual
> privacy, liberty, and protection against discrimination.
> Human rights obligations stemming from the right to health
> care, to social assistance, or from the necessity to improve the
> enjoyment of human rights through international co-operation
> have been neglected. (*AIDS in the World*)

Civil society, the intricate network of shared rights and responsibilities, of social contracts and the integrity of persons, the customs and ways which make a people and a culture, is a living entity. Century-slow beings rise out of time and human interaction, each with its own peculiar vitality. A civil society is a being made by countless individuals, past and present. It lives in that most fragile of abodes, the collective hearts of a populace, in memory, presence, and hope. Precisely because it is so much the creation of a people, civil culture is at once beautifully resilient and deeply vulnerable. A functioning civil society is something like an old-growth forest, full of hidden networks and balances, sustainable and generative. Because the maintenance of civility requires human input, it is perhaps more a garden than a forest, a garden that requires constant care to bring out the inherent beauty of its plantings, and to create spaces of peace, reflection, and inspiration. Like a garden, civil culture too has its wild untended corners, its secret places, secluded corners for lovers and sunlit benches for the old. A Pol Pot, a Ne Win with a band of thugs, an army of Red Guards, can devastate the exquisite gardens of a people with frightening speed and consequences. Sarajevo was once a model of what the Balkans might become: multi-ethnic, sophisticated, tolerant, handsome.

Nowhere is the death of a civil culture more jarring than in China today. What the 11-year Cultural Revolution did not destroy is now threatened by a drive for wealth so intense that you literally choke on its fumes. And this in China, where the orientation of man to his culture and fellows evolved into a kind of secular faith in humanity, ripened over three millennia of carefully recorded history. You see the destruction of civil culture everywhere in the Middle Kingdom, in the garishness of modern Chinese 'traditional' arts (historical references as kitsch, greeting-card Buddhas, hopelessly tacky dragons festooning every overworked surface), the crudeness of social interaction, the brutality of its politics, the suppression of ideas, and the degradation of the environment. Yet China looks sane and functional when compared with Burma and Cambodia, where civil society is still a shambles.

Burma and Cambodia have no common border. What they do share, in addition to ancient, profound Buddhist traditions and past periods of great cultural achievement, are political cultures marked by state violence and corruption, chronic civil war and insurgency, and explosive recent epidemics of HIV infection. It seems almost unbearable that the peoples of these troubled lands should have to face yet another lethal set of obstacles to peace, national reconciliation, and health. But an examination of global HIV/AIDS epidemiology in the developing world suggests that their situations may be not atypical. Uganda in the recent past could be used to make the same argument, as could Haiti under the chaotic military rule of General Cedras; these are countries that have shared the misfortune of having HIV ravage their populations during periods of civil strife under incompetent governments, when civil society was profoundly endangered.

There is no doubt that promotion of condom use is a more direct intervention target than, say, the ending of a simmering insurgency or the establishment of a free press. However, it is perhaps also true that without some measure of social stability and respect for human rights and freedoms, targeted interventions of the sort currently being promoted (condom use, access to antiviral drugs, better STD care, HIV education for youths) may not be sustainable. This is particularly true for prevention programs aimed at women, who universally suffer most when the civic order is chaotic and violent. Such programs may have more problematic consequences as well.

Foreign aid, development assistance, and technical support have all been necessary to help poor countries contend with HIV/AIDS.

These programs, however, can also serve to support problematic regimes and leaders, principally by lending international legitimacy to regimes in power. Governments whose policies could be argued to have hindered HIV prevention or worsened its spread could include Burma's juntas through 2011, the Ceauşescu regime in Romania, Mobuto Sese Seko's single-party state in DR Congo/Zaire, the AIDS denialist government of Thabo Mbeki in South Africa. Supporting such regimes, and lending them legitimacy through donation of HIV/AIDS moneys, may assist in prolonging the political and social situations that have led to explosive HIV spread. The Burmese juntas actively sought such legitimacy, memorably defending themselves in December 1995 UN hearings on human rights violations in the country by listing the number of international agencies and NGOs collaborating with them on HIV/AIDS programs, among others. Hun Sen is a master at this game – winning a coveted Millennium Development Goal Award from the UN for this HIV program in 2010, and still not allowing political freedoms. While researchers and prevention experts may bear no ill intent, and indeed may struggle to establish ethical standards for their own projects in countries like Cambodia there are larger ethical issues at stake. Burma and Cambodia both lost so many of their health professionals, educators, and civil servants, not simply because of poverty or lack of support for social programs, but through repression, imprisonment, and escape. To support such regimes, particularly, as Aung San Suu Kyi has said, when we ourselves come from countries which tolerate basic freedoms and human rights, is, if we accept this premise, illogical in itself, whatever 'good' we believe we are doing by our presence.

A new paradigm for understanding the relationships of public health problems and political realities may be required if we are to address challenges like the spread of HIV/AIDS in countries in turmoil. While humanitarian assistance and strict ethical standards for international involvement must remain priorities, the integration of human rights and political realities into public health discourses and analyses is needed. For many countries there may be no more essential component of HIV programs than respect for human rights

The interaction of HIV, political instability, and human rights abuses in places like Burma, Cambodia, Zimbabwe, Ukraine, should not be surprising; social resources for public health are limited in these countries even in peacetime; their governments are all too often incompetent, corrupt, or both, and persecution against minority groups, intellectuals, journalists, and educated elites are commonplace. Yet in the now extensive HIV/AIDS literature these political realities are too rarely included in discussions of epidemiology, national vulnerability, or barriers to prevention. We are more likely to be informed that in a war-torn African country (several could be named) lack of male circumcision has facilitated HIV spread than that government censorship has eroded a free press, rape of women is widespread and largely unpunished, or that donor funds for health programs have been squandered by corrupt or inept officials. Measures of risk in the public-health literature typically focus exclusively on the behaviors of individuals, even in settings where social systems are patent obstacles to risk reduction. This is not only a lack of intellectual honesty on the part of the medical community, it is bad science.

The classical unit of analysis in epidemiology has been the individual HIV seroconverter and her or his risks. From the behaviors associated with HIV seroconversion, we deduce trends in risk groups, and, if our studies have enough power, in larger populations. This approach has its strengths (rigor, precision, ease of analysis) but also profound limitations. Epidemiology should, at its best, guide and focus preventive efforts. If political and social factors in a given country hinder prevention efforts or facilitate the spread of HIV, these root causes should logically be part of research efforts and intervention programs. Such factors are seldom considered in publications in the medical literature, those of my group included. If they are not included, countries where epidemic spread of HIV is under way are unlikely to achieve control. Yet the public health community is concerned with human rights, particularly as regards the rights of individuals with HIV/AIDS. The foci of these concerns, however, have traditionally been quite narrow. We have paid considerable attention to the ethics of HIV-testing and counseling, informed consent procedures, discrimination and confidentiality, forced or *de facto* isolation and confinement of HIV infected persons, access to care, and the rights of research subjects. There is a large literature around these issues, and articulated systems of review to ensure ethical and human rights standards are met, particularly in research. This is laudable, and by no means to be diminished in importance. But without a wider examination of the human rights context of public health programs, these parameters may be so narrow as to have little actual impact. In Myanmar until 2011, citizens were denied freedom of speech or assembly, a free press, and the right to vote, to create independent non-governmental organizations, and to criticize the military and its policies. Arbitrary arrest, incarceration without trial, and extra-judicial execution by the military had all been documented. Can the rights of people with AIDS be addressed in any meaningful way without taking into account the wider reality of human rights under this kind of regime? To phrase the question differently: can a political body with such policies be expected either to respect the rights of people with or without HIV/AIDS, or to enact effective HIV/AIDS programs?

Perhaps the position of Archbishop Desmond Tutu during the apartheid struggle in South Africa best illustrates where AIDS researchers and organizations eager to help unfree people find themselves. Tutu opposed the immunization programs UNICEF wanted to mount in the old South Africa. UNICEF's position was that 'children are above politics'. Tutu's was that the apartheid system, not lack of vaccines, was at the root of the disproportionate mortality among black children. Since UNICEF's involvement would give legitimacy to the apartheid government's claims to be 'helping' blacks, it had to be resisted. The test of this stance may not be the absolutist moral position that helping children is always a good, but the more complex reality that anything which sustains evil (even medical aid) may prolong suffering. UNICEF is now active in post-apartheid South Africa. There is at the very least a government in power with some accountability, a government that can be openly challenged in elections if it fails, which was not the case under apartheid, where UNICEF's successes or failures would have been closed to scrutiny.

Human rights and Asian values

Are the human rights enshrined in the UN charter and the Geneva Accords applicable in countries like Burma, Indonesia, Malaysia, Vietnam, and China (all of which have argued that they are not)? Or are they imposed by a hostile West on competitor states who have the right to their own interpretation of human rights, which may radically differ from the 'international standard'? Central to the debate on economic and trade policies and human rights between

Asia and the West has been a focus on 'Traditional Asian Values' as opposed to Western ones. Crudely defined (and it is a crude debate, at best), the discourse posits that the Pacific Rim political systems place collective values over individual freedoms, the right to grow economically over the right to express dissent, and the duties and obligations of fixed and reciprocal Confucian hierarchies over democratic principles, including liberal notions of privacy and individuality. Asian economies are growing in the double digits, so the defenders of these values suggest, because Asians are obedient and thrifty; the family, not the state, insures the elderly and the infirm; long-lasting and stable governments ensure long-term planning. The failures of development schemes in Africa and Central America can be seen, in this rubric, to be failures of *values*, Asian miracles as successful examples of the Asian 'way'. These miracle states have also succeeded, so the argument goes, by active suppression of the 'decadent' aspects of modernity, while favoring culturally appropriate expressions of nationalism. Western leaders and the business community, which perhaps belongs to neither East nor West, have understandably begun to support these notions. The dismantling of government social programs across Europe and the U.S. is being accomplished through accepting these values as a challenge to the West's notions of the role of government and the need to compete. It is only natural that business leaders would find appealing the idea that trade unions should be government-controlled, as in Indonesia and China, or that environmental safeguards should never inhibit economic growth, a situation that has already severely damaged the ecosystems of Taiwan, Thailand, China, and others, and that workers should be poorly paid, as they are almost right across Asia. For governments too, the concept that expensive social programs should be scrapped in favor of 'family values' has its appeal. And what government, East or West, would not like to have its exports delinked from any consideration of health, safety, workers' rights, or environmental impacts? Add an open market in weapons and you have a recipe for unprecedented global economic growth.

This can sound like the blueprint for a new era of global prosperity and free trade, or a deeply threatening scenario which could logically include the destruction of the global environment, the end of workers' rights worldwide, an arms race in Asia, and the acceptance of authoritarian government and corporate irresponsibility as viable alternatives to democracy and the rule of law. While the democratic states of the West will no doubt continue to hold elections, have something like a free press, and maintain some aspects of social programs, the need to compete with countries without these restraints on governments and companies would make real opposition virtually impossible. If market forces and unelected governments alone determine the policies of a country, the rights and choices of citizens will be very much beside the point. This is why, while we should perhaps not expect much challenge to the current flirtation with 'Asian values' from the corporate sector, or from governments in power, we should certainly be hearing from citizens' groups, intellectuals, the media, and others who have an interest in people's rights to determine what kind of country, and what kind of world, they want to live in. But the authoritarian governments (China, Indonesia, Malaysia, Vietnam, and Laos, to name a few) who embrace and promote the concepts of Asian values, do not allow these voices to be heard. The price for dissent in such countries is extraordinarily high. When protests are raised by Western voices, 'neo-colonialism' is invoked, or interference in the internal affairs of a sovereign state.

Aung San Suu Kyi penetrated the moral morass of 'Asian values' with characteristic candor and insight. In a videotaped address to the International Labour Organization in Manila in 1995, she pointed out that the rhetoric of the universal rights of man was a cornerstone of Asia's independence movements at the end of the colonial period. Nehru, Sukarno, her father Aung San, and Bandaranaike of Sri Lanka all insisted that Asians should have the same rights as Europeans, rights that been explicitly denied them under European rule. The new states of the region have enshrined these independence heroes in their pantheons, and invoke their names in the search for legitimacy. These new elites, however, have found colonial-era restrictions on democratic rule, dissent, and basic freedoms too tempting and too profitable to ignore. They now insist that their countries have no tradition of universal values, that these are Western impositions, not the very bases of their respective states. Aung San would shudder in horror to discover that the military he founded has perpetuated colonial harshness while eroding what useful legacies the British did leave behind: educational institutions, basic infrastructure, a working public health system.

Given the chance, the people of Burma did not choose 'Asian values'. In the 1990 elections, and again in 2015, they chose the only voice Burma had for universal human rights, respect for the rights of citizens, and non-violent dissent: the National League for Democracy led by Aung San Suu Kyi. If the people of China, or of Vietnam or Laos, were offered a similar opportunity to choose, would they prefer 'Asian values' over the right to speak and think freely, the right to unionize? Until Asians have the right to vote on the 'Asian values' now promoted by their rulers, we should remain deeply skeptical about what unelected governments tell us their citizens want.

'Asian values' were a cornerstone of the thinking prevalent in the mid-1980s, which argued that Asia was spared an HIV problem because of her conservative mores. The decadent West and uncivilized Africans had 'values' problems, which Asians did not. This thinking has since been shown to have been hopelessly wrong-headed. 'Asian values' and traditions did, in fact, have a significant role to play in HIV, not as protective factors, but as risks. Traditions like prostitution, the trafficking and sale of women, the widespread use of these women by unmarried and married men alike, and the extreme reticence of wives to confront their husbands on these grounds, all served to sharply increase HIV susceptibility across the region during the years of rapid spread. It is these traditions that have led to the ultimate violation of persons: slavery – in the Southeast Asian case, debt-bonded sexual slavery. Is there a clearer violation of the shared values of human beings than sex slavery?

Slavery and forced labor are components of the drug detention centers of China, Vietnam, and Cambodia, which have all been criticized for these practices. They continue in the region – perhaps nowhere more clearly demonstrated than in the enslavement of Rohingya refugees from Burma in the regional fishing, canning, and sex industries. China is another matter; investment continues, and the U.S. has neatly articulated how and why. We have 'delinked' human rights issues from trade issues in our dealings with the world's largest potential consumer market. With this sleight of hand we avoid some very complex realities, and we sell out those 1.3 billion consumers at the speed of the sound-bite. But, like a sound-bite, this is easier said than done; 'delinking' economics and human rights may be structurally impossible, in addition to being ethically obscene.

Trade between states is based, at the simplest level, on the economies of the states involved, and economies do not exist without people and their productivity. The conditions of a people, the ways in which their labor, or the resources of the land on which they live, generate wealth is the basis of any economy, and this is the context wherein human rights exist or are violated. Are the people slaves or free agents? If they are exploited by an elite, is the elite corrupt? Can it be held accountable? Are the people organized? Do they have a say in how their lands are used? Can they vote if they do not want their forest cleared or their river dammed? These are questions that cannot be answered without looking at economics and at rights. When people (take the Burmese, for example, or the Chinese who joined the students during the Tiananmen uprising) attempt to claim their rights, to insist that they have a say in how their country be run, basic economic relationships are inextricable from their other demands. The Chinese and Burmese democracy movements were as much protests against corruption and nepotism as they were movements for improvements in human rights. To then say, as the Clinton administration said in the 1990s, that trade and human rights can be dealt with separately, that prison labor and the murder of activists can be neatly put aside when economic considerations are being discussed, is not only a wrong but an absurdity.

This absurdity is not lost on the elites in question. They have really only one concern: power and the privileges of power. As long as trade is uninterrupted, and investment in the economies under their control moves forward, what incentive is there to alter the conditions of that control? And if those conditions involve forced labor, population transfers, the movement of small farmers off their lands, the clear-cutting of forests, the suppression of dissent, why change any of this (profitable in the short term, if not the long) if investors are willing to go along? So the finance minister of the SLORC, Brigadier-General David Abel, commented after another round of 'denunciations' and 'condemnations in the strongest possible language' of his regime in the UN, that, after all, business was still good and foreign investments moving ahead. And the U.S., loudest of all critics, still went ahead with the single largest infrastructure deal in the country, the Unocal oil and gas pipeline. This makes a mockery of the Burmese people's belief that the West – the U.S. and the UN – cares about their rights.

The same complacency must be easing itself into the minds of China's politburo. They made a symbol of Wang Dan, sentencing him to 11 years in prison on the eve of an Asian summit with the U.S., not to insult Bill Clinton or unnerve Warren Christopher, but to remind their own people that trade and human rights were not connected in the 'New World Order', that they could expect no support from the West: that they were alone.

We should, perhaps, be more honest, if only not to delude the brave civilians facing these utterly ruthless elites. We should say, 'It is up to you to change things; we are only interested in the money your country brings to our country, and in the jobs at home our trade with you will help to generate and sustain. If you can seize the day, do it, but be prepared to continue our trade, or we will see to it that you don't get power.' If we really do care that the tennis shoes we buy are cheap because the hands that made them are in chains, we should not buy the shoes.

The British medical journal *The Lancet* regularly publishes many of the seminal studies in medicine. Under the leadership of its gifted editor, the charismatic British physician Richard Horton, the journal has done innovative work in expanding its writ to include political and social aspects of human health that many biomedical journals resist. This has made Richard a sometimes controversial figure. But for the science of HIV, this has made *The Lancet* an essential read precisely because the epidemic, our responses to it, can't be fully understood without reference to context – to laws and policies – to the human rights violations so many living with the virus endure. From the status of women to drug policy reform – the range required to address the complexity of HIV epidemics also calls for broader and deeper study than is generally possible in a single scientific paper. *The Lancet*'s solution has been to develop special theme issues, generally with three to six full papers, shorter commentaries, and 'calls to action' papers with policy and program recommendations. Some have been country specific – there have been great recent series on health in China and India; some of have been disease specific – a number that I've led have taken on specific communities affected by HIV/AIDS.

I first worked with Richard and his *Lancet* team on a special theme issue on Health and Human Rights, published in 2007. With Richard and senior editor Pam Das, we then worked on special theme issues on HIV among People Who Use Drugs in 2010; among MSM in 2012; Sex Workers in 2014; and HIV and related infections in Prisoners and Detainees in 2016. Each was released at the International AIDS Conference in their year of publication. In 2016 we also published a Johns Hopkins–*Lancet* Commission report – a single, substantially longer report, on Drug Policy and Health, which called for an end to the war on drugs, based on a global review of the health impacts of that long, costly, and unwinnable policy failure.

In 2015, *The Lancet* put out series of linked papers on faith and health. I was asked to write a piece for the Faith and Health issue in what *The Lancet* calls 'The Art of Medicine', essay. Personal, reflective, focused on the provider's experience. Taking a line from poet Alexander Pope, the essay was entitled 'The Proper Study of Mankind'.

> Know then thyself, presume not God to scan ...
> The proper study of Mankind is Man.
> Placed on this isthmus of a middle state,
> A Being darkly wise, and rudely great ...
>
> (Alexander Pope, 'Essay on Man,
> Epistle II', 1734)

The tensions between faith traditions and science, belief and reason, have not lessened as scientific understanding has progressed. Advances in genetics alone, from the sequencing of the human genome (and for that matter, the Neanderthal and Denisovan ones) have not only affirmed the fundamental principles of evolution as the bases of the diversity of life, but also helped clarify our prehistory as a species. In what science has begun to call the Anthropocene Epoch, the Age of Man, we have become dominant players in the fate of the biosphere. Who we are, where our civilizations are going, now affects the future of all life with which we share the earth. Yet rather than accept the enormous responsibility we face for stewardship in the Anthropocene, which will require all of our capacities in thinking, making, and caring, there have been striking assertions of faith against science, including denial of evolution or the evidence for climate change. Is scientific evidence and method inherently in conflict with faith? And if not, can the secular, and arguably atheistic, understandings of current science serve as a basis for lives of service? For spirituality?

In what might be called the Judeo–Christian–Islamic continuum, faith in a single deity is a shared cornerstone. Practicing these faiths has called for belief in a deity, adherence to varied laws and tenets, reverence for the tradition's prophets, and study of sacred scripture held to contain revealed truths. Although some faith beliefs (Eve, the first woman, was made from Adam's rib) reflect the realm of myth, great effort has been made to reconcile revealed scripture with evidence from science. Isaac Newton, among many illustrious scientists, struggled with just this conundrum.

In the Hindu–Buddhist continuum, a quite different orientation toward spiritual life has held. These faith traditions have long included an emphasis on praxis – on meditative or yogic practices aimed at the practitioner's development. The historical Buddha Siddhartha Gautama's great reform in the sixth century BC was to focus that praxis tradition on consciousness, on the human mind itself. His realization was both atheistic and strikingly modern; it is best captured, perhaps, in his last words to his disciples: 'Work out your own salvation with diligence'. When probed in a famous discourse about whether the deities of the Hindu pantheon could be said to exist, he replied that the question was irrelevant. If the deities did exist, they too would have to be born into this world, live ordinary human lives, to work out their salvations on this earth. That working out (in English often rendered realization, enlightenment, or liberation), is seen as the goal for us all. Indeed, the enlightened mind is understood as inherent in all of us, and practice is described as a gradual clearing of the obstacles to a fully realized mind, Buddha Mind, which is regarded as the true nature of human consciousness – however painfully far we find ourselves from its realization.

This empirical tradition of focusing on cognition, on mindfulness, on the mind itself, has no greater exemplar in modern Buddhism than His Holiness the Dalai Lama, who has engaged neuroscientists, psychologists, psychiatrists, and others in dialogues around brain science and Buddhist teachings and practices. His Holiness has reiterated his view that if modern brain science should find anything in Buddhist teaching or practice contradicted by empirical evidence, it is Buddhism that will have to change.

As a young man I found the empirical (and atheistic) aspects of Buddhist practice enormously appealing. It was tonic to not be required to believe anything, or to accept a deity, yet to be welcomed to engage in practice. The Mahayana, or Northern School, with its emphasis on compassion, was the path I chose. Taking refuge, as formally becoming a Buddhist is known, I went to Ladakh in the Indian state of Jammu and Kashmir, in 1982. Good timing, as it turned out, since AIDS was about to explode among gay New Yorkers like myself in the U.S. My friends, lovers, patients, and a beloved partner died from AIDS during this time. The epidemic challenged our community to deal with the four noble truths of Buddhist teaching – the inescapable realities of old age, sickness, suffering, and death – in our youth. Death was present with a terrible certainty in that period before effective antiretroviral therapy. And we lived in an often hostile world that would deny us dignity and, sometimes, grace. Yet what we lived through, again and again in those plague years, was witnessing men and women work out their own salvations with diligence. Compassion, to 'suffer with', took on profound new meanings, as did liberation. There was a pressing imperative to try to reduce the unnecessary suffering of others.

That imperative is at the core of what drives many of us in medicine, nursing, research, and public health. And while the goal of alleviating suffering comes for many from their faith and faith traditions, it can and does also come from utterly secular ones. The physician and poet William Carlos Williams memorably remarked that his experience of delivering babies showed him the absurdity, in his eyes, of the doctrine of original sin. Yet Williams also wrote of his primary care medical practice in Patterson, New Jersey, as a practice, by which he meant both a path to the spirit and in his development as an artist. Like Anton Chekhov, Williams' medical practice opened and kept vibrant a wisdom about humanity which still resonates.

Lay Buddhist practice, like Williams' practice, is not so much an admonition to reduce suffering as a praxis approach towards doing so. How? One example relates to motivation. In Buddhist terms actions are seen as neutral. What makes an action virtuous or not, and so favors a good outcome or a bad one, is the motivation of the actor. If an action is driven by self-serving desires, by ego needs, it is unlikely to lead to good outcomes. If an action is motivated by altruism, by the desire to reduce suffering, it is much more likely to lead to good outcomes. This approach makes it imperative to continually interrogate one's own motivations. To ask oneself, deeply and honestly, what is driving an action we would undertake.

Buddhist practice focuses on cognition, on motivation, but also, as the Zen tradition frames it, on understanding 'the way things are'. The teaching of cause and effect is one aspect of this endeavor. Much of what we deal with in daily life, and in the practice of health care, are effects – the downstream outcomes of actions, behaviors, stresses. Like symptoms, they can be alleviated, but rarely fully resolved if our efforts stop at symptomatology alone. Only by getting to the root causes of suffering, the drivers, can we make real progress. This is perhaps most profoundly true in the social and political realms, in my own field of public health, in which social and structural drivers are increasingly understood – and being addressed – as critical to achieve real gains in health.

Another example is the practice of offering merit. In the many and varied folk practices of Buddhist lands, making merit can take on quite formal (and often lovely) aspects of ritual and rite. Candles, incense, offerings to monks and nuns, flower garlands draped on Buddha images, full moon processions in white. The avoidance of meat, alcohol, sex. But offering merit can also be a meditative practice, the making of an internal mental offering up of the benefits of any action to a greater good. Before an action like teaching, say, or giving a public talk, a mental offering is made such as: 'May those hearing this be inspired in their work. May their hearts and minds further open to compassion. May they be empowered to work harder for those who are suffering.' Taking the time to mindfully offer the merit of acts can clarify intent, sharpen the mind on the task to come, and ask, in all humility, that we become clearer conveyers of our disciplines. Shantideva, the incomparable seventh-century Sanskrit poet, said it this way in *The Bodhisattvacharyavatara*:

Thus by the virtue collected
Through all that I have done
May the pain of every living creature
Be completely cleared away.
May I be the doctor and the medicine
And may I be the nurse
For all sick beings in the world
Until everyone is healed.

The proper study of mankind, as the poet averred, is man. Of each of us, ourselves.

To reduce unnecessary suffering, it has always been an imperative to know oneself. This has perhaps never been of more acute import. As a species we have become an existential threat to the very environment that sustains us. We are engaged in worsening conflicts that are generating vast unnecessary human suffering. And yet we know more about the world, nature, life, the human body, than we have ever known. Science has profound parts to play in this moment of challenge – and as scientists it may be of benefit to interrogate our motivations and focus our actions. Life hangs in the balance. And it is too precious to not give our best to preserve and protect.

23 | CONCLUSION: CONDOMS OR LANDMINES

My humble opinion is that without the commitment of leadership at the highest level to preventing further spread of AIDS, we will never see the scale of action necessary to address this issue and its social and economic consequences.

AIDS must be viewed as a national development issue. If we present AIDS as a health problem, it will be treated as such. AIDS is not a health problem, it is a behavioral and societal problem – and an urgent national development priority. Today, AIDS remains the most critical threat to the social and economic progress of the region [Asia and the Pacific] – along with environmental degradation.

The leaders of our countries are not taking AIDS seriously enough. I am here today to tell you about my view as the former Prime Minister of a country facing one of the fastest-spreading AIDS epidemics on the planet, in the hope that we can get more leaders to take AIDS more seriously. We need more action! (Anand Panyarachun, former prime minister of Thailand, addressing the Third International Conference on AIDS in Asia and the Pacific, September 21, 1995, Chiang Mai, Thailand)

Prevention works. Treatment works. HIV epidemic control is possible, even in resource-limited settings. Accountable governments and active public programs can reduce the burden of AIDS, increase life spans into the seventies, and reduce unnecessary suffering. Civil strife, repression, human rights abuses, censorship, corruption, and government neglect can make HIV epidemics worse. Government inaction can add the grief and losses of AIDS to people already burdened. The choice for governments, as a Canadian social theorist put it, is between condoms and landmines, investments in life or in death, improved health or increased suffering.

Morality aside, investments in disease prevention and health promotion are also investments in development, as Khun Anand's eloquent speech attests. Investments in landmines may preserve power elites, may prolong the political lives of parties or individuals, but they can never lead to development. They only add to suffering. Countries ultimately have to choose which way they will go, but governments should be held accountable for those choices. Governments and ideologies which by their actions decrease the health of peoples, or fail to sustain it, are failures, as are those that fail to prepare the young for adult life, and those regimes that degrade the sanctity of ordinary human beings. By these criteria there are some glaring political failures in Southeast Asia. It is only logical that theirs should be the countries most affected by HIV. Near the end of the speech excerpted above, Khun Anand suggested that Asian Development Bank support for development should be linked to a country's commitment to HIV prevention. Spending money on condoms would lead to more money for development. This is the kind of approach that could save millions of lives, and could lead to support for real development, which implies empowerment, participation, and liberation, and to real health, which is more than a state of personal well-being: it is a people's achievement, created and sustained by a just society. It is physical, emotional, and *shared*.

Suffering also is shared.

We can do better. We have the tools now. There is no magic bullet for HIV, but there are few magic bullets for anything. What we need are candid, funded, culture-specific prevention and treatment programs. This will still be true if, and when, an HIV vaccine is available. Polio vaccine is cheap and available, yet polio continues to kill and cripple children in Pakistan and Afghanistan.

The choices are clear. We need more action. Wars in the blood can be won.

NOTES

Preface

1 Mr. Brown, a gay man from San Francisco, was living in Berlin when he was cured. He'd been living with HIV for some years, and was on antiviral therapy when he developed an AIDS-related malignancy. This required a bone marrow transplant. Brown's astute German oncologist had been interested in the small number of people who appeared to have genetic resistance to HIV infection – a genetic variation in the code for a key viral binding reception on their white cells known as the (delta) 32 *nef* deletion. Dr Gero Hütter identified a bone marrow donor with this genetic makeup (the gene appears in about 2 percent of northwestern Europeans – and may have been selected for by the thirteenth-century epidemic of the Black Death, bubonic plague, in this ethnic group). The result, after a complex course which may be difficult to replicate, was that Brown's new immune system post-transplant was genetically resistant to HIV, and he was cured of HIV infection. He remains HIV free after some years off therapy – and is still the only confirmed cure. But in medicine, one case, known as an N of 1, can sometimes provide key information for developing more broadly useful approaches. Stay tuned.

2 Truvada is a two drug combination of the antivirals Emtricitabine and Tenofovir. Tenofovir alone has also been shown to work, among injecting drug users in Thailand.

3 The two regions where incidence is rising and the epidemic still in expansion mode are Eastern Europe and Central Asia, and the Middle East and North Africa. Russia and its out of control epidemic is the principal driver of rising rates in Eastern Europe.

1 Coming into the region

1 The project, 'Preparations for AIDS Vaccine Evaluations' or PAVE, was part of an international initiative funded by the U.S. National Institutes of Health. The Thai PAVE was a collaboration between Chiang Mai University, Johns Hopkins University, the Thai Ministry of Public Health, and the Thai Army Medical Corps. Its purpose was to lay the foundation for possible HIV vaccine trials, a process involving the identification and characterization of people at risk of HIV (but uninfected) who might agree to participation in a vaccine trial. Other PAVE sites included several U.S. cities (Philadelphia, Baltimore, San Francisco, Seattle, and Denver), and sites in India, Haiti, Malawi, Uganda, Rwanda, Kenya, and Zimbabwe. My position, through Johns Hopkins, was field director of the Thai PAVE site.

2 The *wai* is the traditional gesture of greeting and respect in Thailand. The hands are placed palms together and raised to the forehead. It is done with a slight bow and wide smile.

3 Incidence refers to new infection or disease in a previously well person. In Fang we followed about 50 HIV-negative men with known 'risk behaviors' like regular use of prostitutes, a history of recent gonorrhea or syphilis, injecting drug use. None of these men became HIV infected in two years of follow up (1993–1995); a result which surprised

us all and which says volumes for the quality of counseling and HIV prevention the Fang staff were doing. But to identify those 50 negative men we had screened many more; over a third were HIV infected. We also tried to study sex workers in Fang; too few were HIV-negative to justify a study there.

2 Thailand

1 The characterization of the Thai HIV epidemic into waves of spread has been adapted from the seminal paper B.G. Weniger, K. Limpakarnjanarat, K. Ungchusak et al., 'The epidemiology of HIV infection and AIDS in Thailand', *AIDS*, 5 (Suppl. 2) (1991): 871–85.

2 An eerily similar War on Drugs was initiated by the newly elected president of the Philippines, Rodrigo Duterte. He too has used a brutal approach – including calling his people to kill drug addicts – and his policy too seems to be popular with a general public concerned about drug use and convinced that the crackdown is targeting criminals. Thai Prime Minister Samak, who succeeded Thaksin, also threatened to kill 'thousands' of drug users. These policies demonstrate that wars on drugs are likely to continue as long as politicians find them politically expedient.

3 Burma

1 With colleagues from UCLA and with the Karen Department of Health and Welfare, we were able to introduce a rapid blood screening algorithm for malaria, hepatitis B and C and HIV to make transfusions in Eastern Burma's conflict zones much safer.

4 Cambodia

1 Others who have achieved this transition from generalized to concentrated include Eritrea and Honduras.

2 Cambodia's UN-monitored elections were won by the royalist FUNCINPEC Party under the leadership of Prince Ranariddh, a son of Prince Norodom Sihanouk. However, the defeated CPP (Cambodian People's Party) under Hun Sen, the leader supported by Vietnam after the fall of the Khmer Rouge in 1978, demanded to be included in the ruling coalition. Hun Sen, a former Khmer Rouge leader himself, had the largest army in Cambodia at the time, and threatened a return to war if he was not given power. The UN capitulated to this demand in an effort to avoid further fighting. The Cambodian people were thus, once again, denied their choice of government. Ranariddh is officially First Prime Minister and Hun Sen the Second, but he is widely regarded as the real power in Cambodia.

3 While this book was first in press, Cambodia's unstable coalition came to a violent end with the coup d'état of Hun Sen in June 1997. First Prime Minister Ranariddh went into exile, and his forces began fighting Hun Sen's in western Cambodia, threatening a return to all-out civil war. The agony of the Khmer people continues.

4 Lang Samnang, 26, and editor of the independent Idea for Cambodia's Children, was shot after months of threats and warnings from the CPP. Three other journalists have been murdered in Cambodia since 1994.

5 The Khmer Rouge insurgency lingered for several more years and came to end soon after the death of Pol Pot, from malaria, in April of 1998. The tribunal to try five of the remaining leaders for the genocide would not start until 2009.

6 Personal communication, Cambodian Women's Development Association.

7 In July 1997, four weeks after Hun Sen's violent coup, Maha Ghosananda

led a peace march through the streets of Phnom Penh to encourage the country's leaders to resolve their political differences without resorting to violence. Reuters estimated that perhaps 1,300 people, led by hundreds of Buddhist monks and nuns, braved the guns to walk with Maha in support of peace.

5 Laos

1 Reports of continued skirmishes with hold-out Hmong forces were reported in 2015, according to the U.S. State Department, suggesting the resistance was still active.

6 Malaysia

1 Prof. Adeeba later succeeded Marina Mahathir as the Chair of the Malaysian AIDS Council.

10 The flesh trade

1 There are no refugee camps for the Shans along the Thai–Burmese border. If Shans come to Thailand they must find work or starve. This is not the case with the Karen, for example, 80,000 of whom live in camps along this border.

11 Military studies

1 For a thorough investigation of this saga, see Randy Shilts's *Conduct Unbecoming: Gays and Lesbians in the U.S. Military* (St. Martins Press, New York, 1993).

2 This law was struck down, and HIV-infected military personnel continued to serve. The 'Don't Ask Don't Tell' policy of the Clinton era allowed LGBT persons to serve in the military, but persecution of these soldiers, sailors, and air force men and women continued until President Obama led the effort to repeal the policy. LGBTQ persons now serve openly in the U.S. military and the data on HIV infections is now

much more based in reality. HIV in the military looks like HIV in the U.S. – most infections are seen in gay and bisexual men, with men of color having higher burdens. Most women in the military with HIV are minority women, and they are significantly more likely to be from the South.

14 The displaced

1 The Karen conflict is winding down in the Myanmar of today. A ceasefire between the Burmese military and the Karen forces has led to substantive negotiations on a lasting peace accord. Also underway, albeit hesitantly, are discussions around integration of the Karen and other ethnic health workforces into the Myanmar health system.

2 One problem we could address, a major concern of Dr Cynthia's, was improving care for women in pregnancy and labor and delivery in the conflict zones. We collaborated with Mae Tao Clinic and the GHAP team at UCLA on a Mobile Obstetrics Medic (MOM) Project funded by the Gates Population Institute at Johns Hopkins.

16 *Chaai Chuay Chaai*

1 The original group included myself, a Dutch graduate student named Jan Willem der Lind van Wijngaarden, who has since gone on to a long career in the region, and our Thai coordinator, Khun Nui, who later died of AIDS.

18 Activists

1 As told to Mr Anthony Niranam.

19 Drug wars and the war on drugs

1 Buying the raw opium crop from these farmers is cheap, orders of magnitude less expensive then trying to intercept processed heroin further

down the pipeline. During the Carter administration the concept of simply buying the Shan opium crop (then it would have cost about U.S.$10 million) was openly discussed. The policy was called 'preemptive purchase' and had been developed by Carter's special advisor on health, Peter Bourne. It was extremely unpopular in some circles, hailed in others. Serious discussion of the plan was terminated when Peter Bourne was photographed, infamously, using cocaine at an official function. He was dismissed from the White House, and the plan went with him. The Wa are still interested, and have been pressing for direct sales of their crops to the U.S. Drug Enforcement Agency (DEA) for the past eight years; they have no interest in supporting addiction in the U.S., and are seeking support for their cause. We are not buying, however, preferring to spend many hundreds of millions more on trying to stop heroin imports after the cartels have the drugs. This outcome is so illogical as to be perverse, but from a policy perspective perhaps unavoidable, and from a DEA perspective, essential to the survival of their expansive law enforcement budgets.

BIBLIOGRAPHY

Preface

GBD 2015 HIV Collaborators, H. Wang, T.M. Wolock, A. Carter, et al., 'Estimates of global, regional, and national incidence, prevalence, and mortality of HIV, 1980–2015: the Global Burden of Disease Study 2015', *The Lancet*, 3(8) (August 2016): e361–e387. www.thelancet.com/hiv.

Rerks-Ngarm, S., P. Pitisuttithum, S. Nitayaphan, et al., 'Vaccination with ALVAC and AIDSVAX to prevent HIV-1 infection in Thailand', *N Engl J Med*, 361 (2009): 2209–20.

U Pandita, *In This Very Life: Liberation Teachings of the Buddha*, Wisdom Publications, Boston, MA, 1992.

UNAIDS, Global AIDS Update 2016. www.unaids.org/en/resources/dcouments/2016/Global-AIDS-update-2016 [Accessed 12/12/2016].

Introduction

Agence France Presse, 'AIDS looms as threat to Asian Economic boom', *Bangkok Post*, Wednesday, August 3, 1994.

AIDSCAP, UNAIDS, Harvard School of Public Health, 'The status and trends of the global HIV/AIDS pandemic', 11th International Conference on AIDS, Vancouver, Satellite Symposium Final Report, July 1996.

Beyrer, C., S.D. Baral, F. van Griensven, et al., 'Global epidemiology of HIV infection in men who have sex with men', *The Lancet*, 380(9839) (July 28, 2012): 367–77.

Beyrer, C., P.S. Sullivan, J. Sanchez, et al., 'A call to action for comprehensive HIV services for men who have sex with men', *The Lancet*, 380(9839) (July 28, 2012): 424–38.

Bond, K.C., D.D. Celentano, S. Phonsophakul, et al., 'Mobility and migration: female commercial sex work and the HIV epidemic in northern Thailand', in G. Herdt (ed.), *Sexual Cultures and Migration in the Era of AIDS: Anthropological and Demographic Perspectives*, Oxford University Press, New York, 1998, 185–215.

Brookmeyer, R. and M. Gail, *AIDS Epidemiology: A Quantitative Approach*, Oxford University Press, New York, 1994.

Brummelhuis, H.T. and G. Herdt (eds), *Culture and Sexual Risk: Anthropologic Perspectives on AIDS*, Gordon & Breach, Amsterdam, 1996.

Cáceres, C.F., A. Borquez, J.D. Klausner, et al., 'Implementation of pre-exposure prophylaxis for human immunodeficiency virus infection: progress and emerging issues in research and policy', *JIAS*, 19(7 (Suppl. 6)) (October 18, 2016): 21108. doi:10.7448/IAS.19.7.21108. PMID: 27760685.

Cartwright, F. *Disease and History*, Dorset Press, New York, 1972.

Mann, J., D. Tarantola and T. Netter, *AIDS in the World*, Harvard University Press, Cambridge, MA, 1992.

Nelson, K.E., D.D. Celentano, S. Eiumtrakul, et al., 'Changes in sexual behavior and a decline in HIV infection among young men in Thailand', *N Engl J Med*, 335 (1996): 279–303.

Osborne, M., *Southeast Asia: An Introduction* (6th edn), Silkworm Books, Bangkok, 1996.

Panyarachun, A., Address to the 3rd International Conference on AIDS in Asia and the Pacific, Chiang Mai, Thailand, September 21, 1995. An excerpt from this speech can be found on p. 000.

Royal Thai Ministry of Public Health, Division of Communicable Disease Control Region 10, HIV Sentinel Surveillance, 1995, Bangkok.

Sittitrai, W., P. Phanuphak, J. Barry, et al., *Thai Sexual Behavior and Risk of HIV Infection: A Report of the 1990 Survey of Partner Relations and Risk of HIV Infection in Thailand*, Thai Red Cross Society and Chulalongkorn University Press, Bangkok, 1992.

Viravaidya, M., S.A. Obremsky and C. Myers, 'The economic impact of AIDS on Thailand', in *The Economic Implications of AIDS in Asia*, UNDP Publications, New Delhi, 1993.

Way, P.O. and K. Stanecki, 'The demographic impact of an AIDS epidemic on an African country: application of the JWGAIDS model', Center for International Research, Staff paper 58, U.S. Bureau of the Census, Washington D.C., 1991.

Zinsser, H., *Rats, Lice and History*, Little, Brown, Boston, MA, 1934.

2 Thailand

Ainsworth, M., C. Beyrer and A. Soucat, 'Success and new challenges for AIDS control in Thailand', *AIDScience*, 1(5) (2001): 1–5.

Ainsworth, M., C. Beyrer and A. Soucat, 'AIDS and public policy: the lessons and challenges of "success" in Thailand', *Health Policy*, 64(1) (April 2003): 13–37.

Beyrer, C., 'The Kingdom of Lanna and the HIV epidemic', *Journal of The Siam Society*, 83(1–2) (1995): 221–30.

Celentano, D., K. Nelson, S. Suprasert, et al., 'Behavioral and socio-demographic risks for frequent visits to commercial sex workers among northern Thai men', *AIDS*, 7 (1993): 1646–52.

Coedes, G., *The Indianized States of Southeast Asia*, University of Hawai'i Press, Honolulu, HI, 1973.

Ekachai, S., Presentation at Women and AIDS in Thailand Symposium, Chiang Mai, 1993.

Hanenberg, R., W. Rojanapithayakorn, P. Kunasol, et al., 'Impact of Thailand's HIV-control programme as indicated by the decline of sexually transmitted diseases', *The Lancet*, 344 (1994): 243–5.

Havlir, D. and C. Beyrer, 'The beginning of the end of AIDS?', *N Engl J Med* (July 18, 2012). PMID: 22809362.

Head, Jonathan, 'Thailand's bloody drug war', BBC News, February 24, 2003. http://news.bbc.co.uk/go/pr/fr/-/2/hi/asia-pacific/2793763.stm.

Human Rights Watch / Thailand, 'Not enough graves: the war on drugs, HIV/AIDS, and violations of human rights', *Human Rights Watch*, 16(8) (June 2004).

Kitayaporn, D., S. Tansuphaswadikul, P. Lohsomboon, et al., 'Survival of AIDS patients in the emerging epidemic in Bangkok, Thailand', *Journal of AIDS and Human Retrovirology*, 2 (1996): 77–82.

Kunanusont, C., H.M. Foy, J.K. Kreiss, et al., 'HIV-1 subtypes and male-to-female transmission in Thailand', *The Lancet*, 345 (1995): 1078–83.

Kunawararak, P., C. Beyrer, C. Natpratan, et al., 'The epidemiology of HIV and syphilis among male commercial sex workers in northern Thailand', *AIDS*, 9 (1995): 171–6.

Limonanda, B., 'Female commercial sex workers and AIDS: perspectives from Thai rural communities', Fifth

International Conference on Thai Studies, University of London, 1993.

Mastro, T.M. and K. Limpakarnjanarat, 'Condom use in Thailand: how much is it slowing the HIV/AIDS epidemic?', *AIDS*, 9 (1995): 523–5.

McCutchan, F., 'HIV genetic diversity', plenary address at the 9th International Conference on AIDS, Vancouver, 1996.

Muecke, M., 'Mother sold food, daughter sells her body: the cultural continuity of prostitution', *Social Science and Medicine*, 35 (1992): 891–6.

Nelson, K., D. Celentano, S. Suprasert, et al., 'Risk factors for HIV infection among young adult men in northern Thailand', *JAMA*, 270 (1993): 955–60.

Nelson, K.E., V. Suriyanon, E. Taylor, et al., 'The incidence of HIV-1 infections in village populations of northern Thailand', *AIDS*, 8 (1994): 951–5.

Nopkesorn, T., T. Mastro, S. Sangkharomya, et al., 'HIV-1 infection in young men in northern Thailand', *AIDS*, 7 (1993): 1233–9.

Ou, C.-Y., Y. Takebe, C.-C. Lou, et al., 'Wide distribution of two subtypes of HIV-1 in Thailand', *AIDS Research and Human Retroviruses*, 8 (1992) 1471–2.

Rerks-Ngarm, S., P. Pitisuttithum, S. Nitayaphan, et al., 'Vaccination with ALVAC and AIDSVAX to prevent HIV-1 infection in Thailand', *N Engl J Med*, 361 (2009): 2209–20.

Reynolds, C.J. (ed.), *National Identity and Its Defenders: Thailand 1939–1989*, Silkworm Books, Bangkok, 1991.

Royal Thai Ministry of Public Health, Division of Communicable Disease Control HIV/AIDS Surveillance Data, Bangkok, 1995.

Sawanpanyalert, P., K. Ungshusak, S. Thanprasertsuk, et al., 'HIV-1 seroconversion rates among female commercial sex workers, Chiang Mai, Thailand: a multi cross-sectional study', *AIDS*, 8 (1994): 825–9.

Siraprapasiri, J., S. Thanprasertsuk, A. Rodklay, et al., 'Risk factors for HIV among prostitutes in Chiang Mai, Thailand', *AIDS*, 5 (1991): 579–82.

Thienkrua, W., C.S. Todd, W. Chonwattana, et al., 'Incidence of and temporal relationships between HIV, herpes simplex II virus, and syphilis among men who have sex with men in Bangkok, Thailand: an observational cohort', *BMC Infect Dis*, 16 (July 22, 2016): 340. doi:10.1186/s12879-016-1667-z.

Ungphakorn, J. and W Sittitrai, 'The Thai response to the HIV/AIDS epidemic', *AIDS*, 8 (Suppl. 2) (1994): S155–63.

van Griensven, F., T.H. Holtz, W. Thienkrua, et al., 'Temporal trends in HIV-1 incidence and risk behaviours in men who have sex with men in Bangkok, Thailand, 2006–13: an observational study', *The Lancet HIV*, 2(2) (February 2015): e64–e70. doi:10.1016/S2352-3018(14)00031-9. Epub 2015 Jan 8. PMID: 26424462.

Weniger, B.G., K. Limpakarnjanarat, K. Ungchusak, et al., 'The epidemiology of HIV infection and AIDS in Thailand', *AIDS*, 5 (Suppl. 2) (1991): S71–85.

Weniger, B.G., Y. Takebe, C.-Y. Ou, et al., 'The molecular epidemiology of HIV in Asia', *AIDS*, 8 (Suppl. 2) (1994): S13–28.

Wright, J.J., *The Balancing Act*, Asia Books, Bangkok, 1991.

Wyatt, D.K., *Thailand: A Short History*, Yale University Press, New Haven, CT, 1984.

3 Burma

Amnesty International, 'Myanmar: conditions in prisons and labour camps', ASA 16/22/95, London, September 1995.

Aung San Suu Kyi, *Freedom from Fear*, Penguin Books, London, 1991.

Beyrer, C., 'Burma and the challenge of humanitarian assistance', *The Lancet*, 370(9597) (October 27, 2007): 1465–7.

Beyrer, C., M.H. Razak, A. Labrique, et al., 'Assessing the magnitude of the HIV/AIDS epidemic in Burma', *J AIDS*, 32 (2003): 311–17.

Beyrer, C., V. Suwanvanichkij, L. Mullany, et al., 'Responding to AIDS, tuberculosis, malaria and emerging infectious diseases in Burma: dilemmas of policy and practice', *PLoS Med*, 3(10) (October 10, 2006): e393, doi:10.1371/journal.pmed0030393.

Boston Globe, editorial, 'Burma's heroin deal', Boston, November 27, 1996.

Boucaud, A. and L. Boucaud, *Burma's Golden Triangle*, Asia Books, Bangkok, 1992.

Brown, T., 'HIV and AIDS in Asia: Japan conference review', *AIDS Care*, 7(1) (1995): 71–6.

Department of Health, Yangon, 'Annual Report of the AIDS Prevention and Control Programme, Myanmar 1994', Disease Control Programme, Yangon, 1995.

Federation of Trade Unions–Burma, 'Government hospital staff conditions in Burma', presentation at the First HIV/AIDS Policy Forum on Burma, 1996.

Htoon, M.T., H.H. San, K.O. Lwin, et al., 'HIV/AIDS situation in Myanmar', *AIDS*, 8 (Suppl. 2) (1994): S105–9.

Human Rights Watch / Asia, 'Human rights in Burma in 1991', *Human Rights Watch*, 4(24) (1992).

Isett, S., 'Burma's victims of apathy', *Bangkok Post*, September 16, 1994, 36.

Lintner, B., *Outrage*, White Lotus, Bangkok, 1994.

Lintner, B., *Burma in Revolt: Opium and Insurgency since 1948*, White Lotus, Bangkok, 1995.

National Coalition Government of the Union of Burma, *Burma: Human Rights Yearbook, 1995*, NCGUB Press, Bangkok, 1995.

Reuters, 'Khun Sa thrives after rebuilding empire', *Bangkok Post*, January 4, 1997, A2.

Smith, M., *Burma: Insurgency and the Politics of Ethnicity*, Zed Books, London, 1993.

Smith, M., *Fatal Silence: Freedom of Expression and the Right to Health in Burma*, Article 19, London, 1996.

Soe, S., P.P. Win, A.K. Zaw, et al., 'Some characteristics of hospitalized HIV seropositive patients in Myanmar', *Southeast Asian Journal of Tropical Medicine & Public Health*, 24(1) (1993): 18–22.

Southeast Asian Information Network, *Out of Control: The HIV/ AIDS Epidemic in Burma*, SAIN, Chiang Mai, 1995.

Stimson, G., 'HIV infection and injecting drug use in the Union of Myanmar', United Nations International Drug Control Programme, Vienna, 1994.

Suwanvanichkij, V., N. Murakami, C. Lee, et al., 'Community-based assessment of human rights in a complex humanitarian emergency: the Emergency Assistance Teams-Burma and Cyclone Nargis', *Conflict and Health*, 4(1) (April 19, 2010): 8.

Thaung, B., K.M. Gyee and B. Kywe, 'Rapid assessment study of drug abuse in Myanmar: a Ministry of Health and UNDCP co-sponsored project', 9th International Conference on AIDS, Vancouver, Abstract Tu.C.2547, 1996.

Ti, T., H. Naing, P. Noe, et al., 'HIV seroprevalence study in patients attending Union Tuberculosis Institute, Yangon (1994, November and December)', 3rd International Conference on AIDS in Asia and the Pacific, Chiang Mai, Abstract PB128, 1995.

UNICEF, 'Possibilities for a United Nations Peace and Development

Initiative for Myanmar', Unpublished Draft for Consultation, Rangoon, 1992.

Yokota, Y., 'Report on the situation of human rights in Myanmar, prepared by the Special Rapporteur, Mr. Yozo Yokota, in accordance with Commission resolution 1995/72', United Nations, Geneva, 1996. (The reply of the junta to Yokota's charges also makes interesting reading: 'State Law and Order Restoration Council response to the report of the Special Rapporteur, Mr. Yozo Yokota, in accordance with Commission resolution 1995/72', United Nations, Geneva, 1996.)

4 Cambodia

Anon., 'Cambodia returnees bring home HIV', *AIDS Weekly*, India, September 20, 1993, 12–13.

Anon., 'AIDS a bigger danger to army than Khmer Rouge', *Bangkok Post*, July 17, 1995, A3.

Anon., 'AIDS threatens future of Cambodia's military', *The Nation*, Bangkok, July 18, 1996, 1.

Artenstein, A.W., J. Coppola, A.E. Brown, et al., 'Multiple introductions of HIV-1 subtype E into the Western Hemisphere', *The Lancet*, 346 (1995): 1198–9.

Bedford, M., 'Cambodia: still waiting for peace', in *Indochina Interchange*, Oxfam, Boston, MA, 1995.

Beyrer, C., 'Burma and Cambodia: human rights, social disruption, and the spread of HIV/AIDS', *Health and Human Rights*, 2(4) 1998: 84–97.

Brodine, S.K., J.R. Mascola, P.J. Weiss, et al., 'Detection of diverse HIV-1 subtypes in the United States', *The Lancet*, 346 (1995): 1199–200.

Cambodian Human Rights Foundation, 'Rapid appraisal of the human rights vigilance of Cambodia on child prostitution and trafficking, March–April 1995', CHRF, Phnom Penh, 1995.

Cambodian Women's Development Association, 'Prostitution and traffic of women: a dialogue on the Cambodian situation', CWDA Special Reports, Phnom Penh, 1996.

Chandler, D.P., *A History of Cambodia* (2nd edn), Westview, Boulder, CO, 1993.

Chang, P.M., *Kampuchea between China and Vietnam*, Singapore University Press, Singapore, 1987.

Chanthou, B., 'Grim picture of women's lot', *Phnom Penh Post*, Phnom Penh, June 1, 1995.

Chhi Vun, M., M. Fujita, T. Rathavy, et al., 'Achieving universal access and moving towards elimination of new HIV infections in Cambodia', *JIAS*, 17 (2014): 18905.

Davies, J. 'HIV rates among MSM stubbornly high: study', *Phnom Penh Post*, November 16, 2016.

Escoffier, C., 'Sexually transmitted diseases in Banteay Meanchey [Cambodia]', Médecins Sans Frontières, 1995.

Ghosananda, M., *Step by Step*, Parallax Press, Berkeley, CA, 1992.

Kongkea, R., 'IDS victims on the rise', *Phnom Penh Post*, Phnom Penh, April 3, 1996.

Land-Mines Advisory Group, Information on the landmine situation in Cambodia was kindly provided to the author by staff of the Land-Mines Advisory Group, Phnom Penh, 1996.

Page, K., E, Stein, N. Sansothy, et al., 'Sex work and HIV in Cambodia: trajectories of risk and disease in two cohorts of high-risk young women in Phnom Penh, Cambodia', *BMJ Open*, 3(9) (2013): e003095. doi:10.1136/bmjopen-2013-003095.

Reuters, 'Japanese troops get AIDS virus in Cambodia', *Sankei Shimbun*, Tokyo, October 20, 1993, 1.

Reuters, 'Cambodian editor wounded in shooting', *Bangkok Post*, January 4, 1997, A2.

Saddhatissa, H. (ed.), *Sutta Nipata*, Salem House, Cambridge, MA, 1985.

Sherry, A., M. Lee and M. Vatikiotis, 'For lust or money', *Far Eastern Economic Review*, 3 (1995): 22–3.

Tia, P., et al., 'The epidemiology of HIV in Cambodia', 10th International Conference on AIDS, Yokohama, abstract PC0621, 1994.

U.S. Department of State, Human Rights Report, *Cambodia*, 2015.

Yi, S., S. Tuot, P. Chhoun, et al., 'Factors associated with recent HIV testing among high-risk men who have sex with men: a cross-sectional study in Cambodia', *BMC Public Health*, 15 (2015): 743.

5 Laos

Chan, S. (ed.), *Hmong Means Free*, Temple University Press, Philadelphia, PA, 1994.

Dammen, A.J., *Laos: Keystone of Indochina*, Westview, London, 1985.

Finch, P. and S. Chantavanich (eds), 'The Lao returnees in the voluntary repatriation programme from Thailand', *Indochina Chronology*, Occasional Papers Series No. 03, Indochinese Refugee Information Center, January–March, 1995.

GBD 2015 HIV Collaborators, H. Wang, T.M. Wolock, A. Carter, et al., 'Estimates of global, regional, and national incidence, prevalence, and mortality of HIV, 1980–2015: the Global Burden of Disease Study 2015', *The Lancet*, 3(8) (August 2016): e361–e387. www.thelancet.com/hiv.

Gunn, C.G., *Rebellion in Laos: Peasant and Politics in a Colonial Backwater*, Westview, Boulder, CO, 1990.

Hamilton-Merritt, J., *Tragic Mountains: The Hmong, the Americans, and the Secret Wars far Laos, 1942–1992,* Indiana University Press, Indianapolis, IN, 1993.

Lintner, B., *Outrage*, White Lotus, Bangkok, 1994.

Lintner, B., *Burma: Opium and Insurgency since 1948*, White Lotus, Bangkok, 1995.

McCoy, A.W., *The Politics of Heroin in Southeast Asia*, HarperCollins, New York, 1972.

Prasongsith, B.C., P. Blanche, K. Phouvang, et al., 'HIV infection in Lao Republic', 10th International Conference on AIDS, Yokohama, 1994.

6 Malaysia

Anti-Narcotics Task Force, Malaysia, 'Malaysia Narcotics Report 1994', National Security Council, Prime Minister's Department, Kuala Lumpur, 1994.

Asia Watch, *A Modern Form of Slavery: Trafficking of Burmese Women and Girls into Brothels in Thailand*, Asia Watch/Human Rights Watch, Bangkok, 1993.

Beyrer, C., K.P. Ng, T. Van Cott, et al., 'Short communication: HIV-1 subtypes in Malaysia, determined with serologic assays: 1992–1996', *AIDS Research and Human Retroviruses*, 14(18) (1997): 1687–91.

Brown, T.M., K.E. Robbins, M. Sinniah, et al., 'HIV Type 1 subtypes in Malaysia include B, C, and E', *AIDS Research and Human Retroviruses*, 12(17) (1996): 1655–7.

East-West Center, *AIDS in Asia: The Gathering Storm*, University of Hawai'i, Honolulu, HI, 1994.

Lam, S.K., 'HIV and AIDS: the road ahead', proceedings of Workshop on the Epidemiology of HIV and AIDS, Kuala Lumpur, 1996.

Limonanda, B., 'Demographic and behavioral study of female commercial sex workers in Thailand',

Special Report, Institute of Population Studies, Chulalongkorn University, Bangkok, 1993.

Limonanda, B., G.S.D. van Griensven, N. Changvatana, et al., 'Condom use and risk factors for HIV-1 infection among female commercial sex workers in Thailand', *American Journal of Public Health*, 84 (1994): 2026–7.

Ministry of Health, Malaysia, *Reporting of HIV/AIDS in Malaysia*, AIDS/STD Section, Kuala Lumpur, 1996.

Ministry of Health, Malaysia, *Malaysia 2015: Country Responses to HIV/ AIDS*, Ministry of Health, Malaysia, December, 2014.

Rahman, F. and A. Kamarulzaman, 'Southeast Asia in focus: stemming the reawakening of prohibitionism', *JIAS*, 19 (2016): 21279. http://dx.doi. org/10.7448/IAS.19.1.21279.

Royal Thai Ministry of Public Health, Division of Communicable Disease Control, HIV/AIDS Surveillance Data, Bangkok, 1995.

Singh, J., S. Che'Rus, S. Chong, et al., 'AIDS in Malaysia', *AIDS*, 8 (Suppl. 2) (1994): S99–103.

Sittitrai, W., *The Sun*, Kuala Lumpur, Malaysia, July 19, 1995, 8.

Teoh Bing Fei J., A. Yee, M.H. Habil, et al., 'Effectiveness of methadone maintenance therapy and improvement in quality of life following a decade of implementation', *J Subst Abuse Treat*, 69 (October 2016): 50–56. doi:10.1016/j.jsat.2016.07.006.

Tsuchide, H., T.S. Saraswathy, M. Sinniah, et al., 'HIV-1 variants in South and South-East Asia', *International Journal of STD and AIDS*, 6 (1995): 117–220.

7 Vietnam

Berry, M.C., V.F. Go, V.M. Quan, et al., 'Social environment and HIV risk among MSM in Hanoi and Thai Nguyen', *AIDS Care*, 25(1) (2013): 38–42.

CARE International Vietnam, 'An audience analysis of urban men and sex workers', Special Report, CARE, Hanoi, 1993.

CARE International Vietnam, 'Targeting young men: AIDS prevention in Vietnam', Special Report, CARE, Hanoi, 1994.

CDC in Vietnam, Fact Sheet, 2016.

Colby, D., N.A Nguyen, B. Le, et al., 'HIV and syphilis prevalence among transgender women in Ho Chi Minh City, Vietnam', *AIDS Behav*, 20 (Suppl. 3) (2016): 379–85.

Franklin, B. and I. Brugemann, 'Women and the risk of HIV/AIDS in Vietnam', *AIDS Analysis Asia*, 4 (1995).

Franklin, B. and N.T. Khanh, 'The fire in the dragon: a study of risk factors for HIV/AIDS among urban men and commercial sex workers in Vietnam', 10th International Conference on AIDS, Yokohama, Abstract 031D, 1984.

Huong, N.D., 'Tuberculosis and HIV infection in Vietnam', 3rd International Conference on AIDS in Asia and the Pacific, Chiang Mai, Abstract PB127, 1995.

Kahane, T., 'Turning the tide', *Asia Week*, April 10, 1996.

Ministry of Health, Vietnam, *Report of the National AIDS Control Committee*, Hanoi, 1995.

Nguyen, N.N.T. and T.O. Nguyen, *Will to Live: An Oral History of Five People Who Are Found to be HIV-Positive*, CARE International in Vietnam, Hanoi, 1995.

Sheehan, N., *Two Cities: Hanoi and Saigon*, Jonathan Cape, London, 1992.

UNAIDS, 'The status and trends of the global HIV/AIDS pandemic', 11th International Conference on AIDS, Vancouver, Satellite Symposium Final Report, Geneva, 1996.

Vietnam News, 'HIV response must cover women', Update February 2016.

Windle, J. *A Slow March from Social Evil to Harm Reduction: Drugs and Drug Policy in Vietnam*, Center for 21st Century Security and Intelligence Latin America Initiative, Improving Global Drug Policy: Comparative Perspectives and UNGASS 2016, Brookings Institution, 2016.

8 Yunnan

Beyrer, C., 'HIV/AIDS in Asia: accelerating and disseminating', *The Washington Quarterly*, 24(1) (2000): 211–25.

Beyrer, C., 'Hidden epidemic of sexually transmitted diseases in China: crisis and opportunity', *JAMA*, 298(10) (2003): 1303–5.

Beyrer, C., 'An epidemic of denial: stalled responses to HIV/AIDS in China', *Harvard Intern'l Rev*, 25(2) (2003): 64–8.

Beyrer, C., M.H. Razak, K. Lisam, et al., 'Overland heroin trafficking routes and HIV spread in South and Southeast Asia', *AIDS*, 14 (2000): 1–9.

Chin, J., 'Scenarios for the AIDS epidemic in Asia', *Asia-Pacific Population Research Reports*, 2 (1995).

Chuang, C.-Y., P.-Y. Chang and K.-C. Lin, 'AIDS in the Republic of China', *Clinical Infectious Diseases*, 17 (Suppl. 2) (1993): S337–40.

Cowley, G., 'China: when AIDS finally hits', *Newsweek*, April 15, 1996.

Department of Disease Control, Ministry of Health, *AIDS Prevention and Control in China*, China Pictorial Publishing House, Beijing, 1994.

Lintner, B., *Burma in Revolt: Opium and Insurgency since 1948*, White Lotus, Bangkok, 1995. (Contains some fascinating historical information on the origins of the modern drug routes in the region.)

McCutchan, F.E., J.K. Carr, D. Murphy, et al., 'Precise mapping of recombination breakpoints suggests a common parent of two BC recombinant HIV type 1 strains circulating in China', *AIDS Research and Human Retroviruses*, 18(15) (October 10, 2002): 1135–40.

Piriyasilip, S., F. McCutchan, J.K. Carr, et al., 'A recent outbreak of HIV-1 infection in southern China was initiated by two highly homogenous, geographically separated strains: circulating recombinant for AE and a novel BC recombinant', *J Virology*, 74(23) (2000): 11286–95.

Spartacus, *Spartacus International Gay Guide*, Bruno Gmunder, Berlin, 1995–1996.

Tyler, P.E., 'Heroin influx ignites a growing AIDS epidemic in China', *New York Times*, November 28, 1995.

Wan Yanhai and Li Xiarong, 'Consequences of a stalled response: iatrogenc epidemic among blood donors in central China', in C. Beyrer and H. Pizer (eds), *Public Health and Human Rights: Evidence-Based Approaches*, Johns Hopkins University Press, Baltimore, MD, 2007, 65–87.

Yu, E.S.H., X. Qiyi, Z. Konglai, et al., 'HIV infection and AIDS in China, 1985–1994', *American Journal of Public Health*, 86 (1996): 1116–22.

Yu, X.F., J. Chen, Y. Shao, et al., 'Two subtypes of HIV-1 among injection-drug users in southern China [Letter]', *The Lancet*, 351(9111) (1998): 1250.

Yu, X.F., J. Chen, Y. Shao, et al., 'Emerging HIV infections with distinct subtypes of HIV-1 among injection drug users from geographically separated locations in Guangxi Province, China', *J AIDS*, 22 (1999): 180–88.

Zeng Yi, 'The working situation of controlling and preventing AIDS in China', presentation at the International Symposium on AIDS, Beijing, China, 1995.

Zunyou Wu, R. Detels, Jiangpeng Zhang, et al., 'Risk factors for intravenous drug use and sharing of equipment among young male drug users in southwest China', presentation at the International Symposium on AIDS, Beijing, China, 1995.

9 Women

Anon., 'Bringing AZT to poor countries', *Science*, 269(4) (1995): 624–5.

Brown, T., W. Sittitrai, S. Vanichseni, et al., 'The recent epidemiology of HIV and AIDS in Thailand', *AIDS*, 8 (Suppl. 2) (1994): S131–41.

Burton, R. (trans.), in A.H. Walton (ed.), *The Perfumed Garden of the Shaykh Nefzawi*, Gramercy Publishing, New York, 1964.

Cohen, M.S., Y.Q. Chen, M. McCauley, et al. (HPTN 052 Study Team), 'Prevention of HIV-1 infection with early antiretroviral therapy', *N Engl J Med*, 365(6) (August 11, 2011): 493–505. doi:10.1056/NEJMoa1105243.

Connor, E.M., R.S. Sperling, R. Gelbert, et al., 'Reduction of maternal-infant transmission of human immunodeficiency virus type I with zidovudine treatment', *N Engl J Med*, 331 (1994): 1173–80.

Elias, C., 'Sexually transmitted diseases and the reproductive health of women in developing countries', The Population Council, Working Paper 5, 1991.

Fleming, P.S., 'Access to treatments in developing countries', address at the 11th International Conference on AIDS, Vancouver, 1996.

Nelson, K.E., D.D. Celentano, S. Eiumtrakul, et al., 'Changes in sexual behavior and a decline in HIV infection among young men in Thailand', *N Engl J Med*, 335 (1996): 279–303.

Wasserheit, J., 'Epidemiologic synergy: interrelationships between human immunodeficiency virus infection and other sexually transmitted diseases', *Sexually Transmitted Diseases*, 19 (1991): 62–4.

For a thorough discussion of heterosexual transmission of HIV, see also I. De Vincenzi (for the European Study Group on Heterosexual Transmission of HIV), 'A longitudinal study of human immunodeficiency virus transmission by heterosexual partners', *N Engl J Med*, 331 (1994): 341–6.

10 The flesh trade

Albert, A.E., D.L. Warner, R.A. Hatcher, et al., 'Condom use among female commercial sex workers in Nevada's legal brothels', *American Journal of Public Health*, 85 (1995): 1514–20.

Baral, S., C. Beyrer, K. Muessig, et al., 'Burden of HIV among female sex workers in low-income and middle-income countries: a systematic review and meta-analysis', *The Lancet Infect Dis*, D-12-00060, March 15, 2012.

Cambodian Women's Development Association, Mission Statement, 1995.

Cambodian Women's Development Association, 'Prostitution and traffic of women and children', conference report, Phnom Penh, 1995.

Decker, M.R., A.L. Crago, S.K. Chu, et al., 'Human rights violations against sex workers: burden and effect on HIV', *The Lancet*, (July 21, 2014). pii:S0140-6736(14)60800-X. doi:10.1016/S0140-6736(14)60800-X.

Downs, A.M. and I. De Vincenzi, 'Probability of heterosexual transmission of HIV: relationship to the number of unprotected sexual contacts', *Journal of AIDS and Human Retrovirology*, 11 (1996): 388–95.

Estebanez, P., K. Fitch and R. Najera, 'HIV and female sex workers', *Bulletin of the World Health Organization*, 71(3/4) (1993): 397–412.

Fairclough, G., 'Doing the dirty work: Asia's brothels thrive on migrant labour', *Far Eastern Economic Review*, December 14, 1995, 27–8.

Federation of Trade Unions–Burma, 'A survey of the HIV/AIDS and migrant workers situation in Ranong', *FTUB Special Report*, Washington, D.C., 1996.

Holthausen, J., 'Burma's AIDS crisis', *Het Parool*, December 1, 1996, A1 (in Dutch).

Hunt, C., 'Migrant labor and sexually transmitted disease: AIDS in Africa', *Journal of Health and Human Behavior*, 30 (1989): 353–73.

Institute of Population Studies, Chulalongkorn University, 'Surveys of commercial sex workers in Sugai Kolok, Narathiwat Province and Batong, Vala Province, 1994', presentation at the Consultation on Information and Population Movement and HIV/AIDS, Bangkok, Thailand, 1996.

Masenior, N. and C. Beyrer, 'The U.S. Anti-Prostitution Pledge: First Amendment challenges and public health priorities', *PLoS Med*, 4(7) (July 24, 2007): e207.

Mastro, T.M., G.A. Satten, T. Nopkesorn, et al., 'Probability of female-to-male transmission of HIV-1 in Thailand', *The Lancet*, 343 (1994): 204–7.

McKeganey, N.P., 'Prostitution and HIV: what do we know and where might research be targeted in the future?', *AIDS*, 8 (1994): 1215–26.

Plummer, F.A., K. Fowke, N.J.D. Nagelkerke, et al., 'Resistance to HIV among continuously exposed prostitutes in Nairobi', 11th International Conference on AIDS, Berlin, Abstract WS-A07-3, 1993.

Pollock, J., 'Migrant workers and discrimination', address at the 1st Policy Forum on Addressing the AIDS Epidemic in Burma, 1996.

Pramaulratana, A., presentation at the 1st Technical Consultation on Migration and AIDS, Asian Institute of Population Studies, Chulalongkorn University, Bangkok, 1995.

Reade, R., G. Richwald and N. Williams, 'The Nevada legal brothel system as a model for AIDS prevention among female sex industry workers', 6th International Conference on AIDS, San Francisco, 1990.

Rowland-Jones, S., J. Sutton, K. Ariyoshi, et al., 'HIV-specific cytotoxic T-cells in HIV-exposed but uninfected Gambian women', *Nature Medicine*, 1 (1995): 59–64.

Royal Thai Ministry of the Interior, quoted by G. Risser, 'Population movements in South-East Asia', Asian Research Center for Migration, Chulalongkorn University, Bangkok, 1994.

Royal Thai Ministry of the Interior, Thai National Labor Statistics, Bangkok, 1995.

Shrey, A., M. Lee and M. Vatiklotis, 'Sex trade: for lust or money', *Far Eastern Economic Review*, December 14, 1995, 22–3.

Strathdee, S.A., A.L. Crago, J. Butler, et al., 'Dispelling myths about sex workers and HIV', *The Lancet*, (July 21, 2014). pii:S0140-6736(14)60980-6. doi:10.1016/S0140-6736(14)60980-6.

United Nations High Commission for Refugees, 'Response to CWDA allegations of UNTAC's role in trafficking in Cambodia', Phnom Penh Conference on Traffic of Women and Children, 1995.

Vanaspong, C., 'Prostitution: new law won't help', *Bangkok Post*, April 7, 1996, 17.

11 Military studies

Altman, L.K., 'After setback, first large AIDS vaccine trials are planned', *New York Times*, November 29, 1994, B6–7.

Anon., 'The profits and losses of AIDS', *The Economist*, July 13, 1996, 81–2.

Anon., 'AIDS threatens future of Cambodia's military', *The Nation*, Bangkok, July 18, 1996, 1.

Celentano, D.D., K. Bond, C. Lyles, et al., 'Preventive intervention to reduce sexually transmitted infections: a field trial in the Royal Thai Army', *Arch Intern Med*, 160 (2000): 535–40.

Levin, L.I., T.A. Peterman, P.O. Renzullo, et al., 'HIV-1 seroconversion and risk behaviors among young men in the US Army', *American Journal of Public Health*, 85 (1995): 1500–506.

Nelson, K.E., D.D. Celentano, S. Eiumtrakul, et al., 'Changes in sexual behavior and a decline in HIV infection among young men in Thailand', *N Engl J Med*, 335 (1996): 297–303.

Nelson, K.E., D.D. Celentano, S. Suprasert, et al., 'Risk factors for HIV infection among young adult men in northern Thailand', *JAMA*, 270(8) (1993): 955–60.

Nelson, K., S. Eiumtrakul, D.D. Celentano, et al., 'HIV infection in young men in Thailand, 1991–1998: increasing role of injection drug use', *J AIDS*, 29 (2002): 62–8.

Rangsin, R., K. Kana, T. Chuenchitra, et al., 'Risk factors for HIV infection among young Thai men during 2005–2009', *PLoS One*, 10(8) (August 26, 2015): e0136555. doi:10.1371/journal.pone.0136555. eCollection 2015.

Shilts, R., *Conduct Unbecoming: Gays and Lesbians in the U.S. Military*, St. Martins Press, New York, 1993.

Thein, M.T., S. Than, B. Kywe, et al., 'Sexual risk behaviors in young soldiers' HIV and VDRL seroprevalence', Department of Defense Medical Services, Myanmar, 3rd International Conference on AIDS in Asia and the Pacific, Chiang Mai, Thailand, Abstract B304, 1995.

Verghese, B.G., *India's Resurgent Northeast: Ethnicity, Insurgency, Governance, Development*, Center for Policy Research, Konark, Delhi, 1996.

12 Chasing the dragon

Celentano, D.D., A. Munoz, S. Cohn, et al., 'Drug-related behavior change for HIV transmission among injection drug users', *Addiction*, 89 (1994): 1309–17.

Choopanya, K., S. Vanichseni, D.C. Des Jarlais, et al., 'Risk factors and HIV seropositivity among injecting drug users in Bangkok', *International Journal of Addictions*, 26 (1991): 1333–47.

Csete, J., A. Kamarulzaman, M. Kazatchkine, et al., 'Public health and international drug policy', *The Lancet*, 387(10026) (April 2, 2016): 1427–80. doi:10.1016/S0140-6736(16)00619-X. Review. PMID: 27021149.

Des Jarlais, D.C., M. Marmor, D. Paono, et al., 'HIV incidence among injecting drug users in New York City syringe exchange programmes', *The Lancet*, 348 (1996): 987–91.

Merson, M., 'Returning home: reflections on the USA's response to the HIV/AIDS epidemic', *The Lancet*, 347 (1996): 1673–6. (This presents a lucid analysis of U.S. prevention policy and its limitations.)

Nelson, K.E., 'The epidemiology of HIV infection among injecting drug users and other risk populations in Thailand', *AIDS*, 8 (1994): 1499–500.

Nelson, K.E., D. Vlahov, S. Cohn, et al., 'Human Immunodeficiency Virus infection in diabetic intravenous drug users', *JAMA*, 266 (1991): 2259–61.

Nyein, Nyein, 'Report links increased militarization and drug trade in eastern Shan State', *The Irrawaddy*, October 27, 2016.

Phanupak, P., V. Posyachinda, T. Uenklabh, et al., 'HIV transmission among intravenous drug abusers', 5th International Conference on AIDS, Montreal, Abstract TG025, 1989.

Shilts, R., *And the Band Played On: Politics, People, and the AIDS Epidemic*, St. Martin's Press, New York, 1987.

United Nations Office on Drugs and Crime, *World Drug Report, 2015*. http://www.unodc.org/wdr2015/.

Vanichseni, S., B. Wongsuwan, K. Choopanya, et al., 'A controlled trial of methadone maintenance in a population of intravenous drug users in Bangkok: implications for prevention of HIV', *International Journal of Addictions*, 26 (1991): 1313–20.

Weniger, B. and T. Brown, 'The march of AIDS through Asia', *N Engl J Med*, 335(5) (1995): 343–4.

Xia, M., J.K. Kreiss and K.K. Holmes, 'Risk factors for HIV infection among drug users in Yunnan Province, China: association with intravenous drug use and protective effect of boiling reusable needles and syringes', 9th International Conference on AIDS, Berlin, Abstract WS-C15-1, 1993.

13 Tribes

Beyrer, C., S. Suprasert, W. Sittitrai, et al., 'Widely varying prevalence and risk behaviors and HIV infection among the hilltribe and ethnic minority peoples of upper northern Thailand', *AIDS Care*, 9(4) (1997): 427–39.

Filbeck, D., 'The Lua of Nan Province', *Journal of the Siam Society*, 77(1) (1989): 102–9.

Gray, J., 'The social and sexual mobility of young women in rural northern Thailand: Khon Muang and hilltribes', paper presented at the 1st Workshop on Sociocultural Dimensions of HIV/AIDS Control and Care in Thailand, Chiang Mai, 1994.

Hamilton, J.W., *Pwo Karen: At the Edge of Mountain and Plain*, West Publishing, St. Paul, MN, 1976.

Kammerer, C.O., O. Klein Hutheesing, R. Maneeprasert, et al., 'Vulnerability to HIV infection among three hill tribes in northern Thailand: qualitative anthropological issues', presentation at the 5th International Conference on Thai Studies, SOAS, London, 1993.

Kammerer, C.O., O. Klein Hutheesing, R. Maneeprasert, et al., 'Vulnerability to HIV infection among three hill tribes in northern Thailand', in H.T. Brummelhuis and G. Herdt (eds), *Culture and Sexual Risk: Anthropologic Perspectives on AIDS*, Gordon & Breach, Amsterdam, 1996, 53–76.

Klein Hutheesing, O., 'Linking the Lisu to the HIV/AIDS epidemic: observations of a cultural-political kind', paper presented at the 1st Workshop on Sociocultural Dimensions of HIV/AIDS Control and Care in Thailand, Chiang Mai, 1994.

Kunstadter, P., 'Cultural factors related to transmission and control of HIV infection: highland minorities of northern Thailand', paper presented at the 1st Workshop on Sociocultural Dimensions of HIV/AIDS Control and Care in Thailand, Chiang Mai, 1994.

Leiter, K., I. Tamm, C. Beyrer, et al., 'No status: migration, trafficking and exploitation of women in Thailand: health and HIV/AIDS risks for Burmese and hill tribe women and girls', *Physicians for Human Rights*,

June 2004; Special Report, Boston, MA.

Lewis, P. and E. Lewis, *Peoples of the Golden Triangle*, Thames and Hudson, London, 1984.

Milne, L., *The Shans at Home*, Paragon Books, New York, 1970.

Symonds, P., 'The political and cultural economy of the Hmong as related to HIV/AIDS: observations from the field', paper presented at the 1st Workshop on Sociocultural Dimensions of HIV/AIDS Control and Care in Thailand, Chiang Mai, 1994.

Thai National Statistics Office, *Summary Report of the Survey of Hilltribes in Thailand, 1985–1988*, Office of the Prime Minister, National Statistics Office in collaboration with the Department of Public Welfare, Bangkok, 1993.

Tribal Research Institute, Chiang Mai University, *A Socio-Cultural Study of the Impact of Social Development Programs on Tribal Women and Children*, Faculty of Social Sciences, Chiang Mai University Press, Chiang Mai, 1985.

Walker, A.R., 'In mountain and "Ulu": a comparative history of development strategies for ethnic minority peoples in Thailand and Malaysia', *Contemporary Southeast Asia*, 4(4) (1983): 451–85.

Yu, E.S.H., X. Qjyi, Z. Konglai, et al., 'HIV infection and AIDS in China, 1985–1994', *American Journal of Public Health*, 86 (1996): 1116–22.

14 The displaced

Beyrer, C., S. Baral and J. Zenilman, 'STDs, HIV/AIDS and migrant populations', in K.K. Holmes, P.F. Sparling, W.E. Stamm, et al. (eds), *Sexually Transmitted Diseases* (4th edn), McGraw Hill, New York, 2007, 257–68.

Beyrer, C., V. Suwanvanichkij, L. Mullany, et al., 'Responding to AIDS, tuberculosis, malaria and emerging infectious diseases in Burma: dilemmas of policy and practice', *PLoS Med*, 3(10) (October 10, 2006): e393. doi:10.1371/journal. pmed0030393.

Davis, W.W., L.C. Mullany, E.K. Shwe Oo, et al., 'Health and human rights in Karen State, eastern Myanmar', *PLoS One*, 10(8) (August 26, 2015): e0133822. doi:10.1371/journal. pone.0133822. eCollection 2015. PMID: 26308850.

Lee, T.J., L.C. Mullany, A. Richards, et al., 'Mortality rates in conflict zones: Karen, Karenni, and Mon states in eastern Burma', *Tropical Medicine and International Health*, 11(7) (July 2006): 1197–227.

Leiter, K., V. Suwanvanichkij, I. Tamm, et al., 'Human rights abuses and vulnerability to HIV/AIDS: the experiences of Burmese women in Thailand', *Health & Human Rights*, 2 (December 2006): 88–111.

Leiter, K., I. Tamm, C. Beyrer, et al., 'No status: migration, trafficking and exploitation of women in Thailand: health and HIV/AIDS risks for Burmese and hill tribe women and girls', *Physicians for Human Rights*, June 2004; Special Report, Boston, MA.

Mullany, L.C., C.I. Lee, P. Paw, et al., 'The MOM Project: efforts to increase access to reproductive services among internally displaced populations in Burma', *Reproductive Health Matters*, 16(31) (May 2008): 44–56.

Mullany, L.C., C. Lee, L. Yone, et al., 'Access to essential maternal health interventions and human rights violations among vulnerable communities in eastern Burma', *PLoS Med*, 5(12) (December 23, 2008): 1689–98.

Mullany, L.C., T.J. Lee, L. Yone, et al., 'Impact of community-based maternal health workers on coverage of essential maternal health interventions among internally displaced communities in eastern Burma: the MOM Project', *PLoS Med*, 7(8) (August 3, 2010): e1000317.

Mullany, L., C. Maung and C. Beyrer, 'HIV/AIDS knowledge, attitudes and practices among Burmese migrant factory workers in Tak Province, Thailand', *AIDS Care*, 15(1) (2003): 63–70.

Teela, K.C., L.C. Mullany, C.I. Lee, et al., 'Community-based maternal health care in conflict-affected areas of eastern Burma: experiences from the field', *Social Science Medicine*, 68(7) (April 2009): 1332–40.

15 Other genders

Anchalee, Thai Lesbian Network, presentation at the Foreign Correspondents Club of Thailand, Bangkok, September 1995.

Baral, S.D., T. Poteat, S. Strömdahl, et al., 'Worldwide burden of HIV in transgender women: a systematic review and meta-analysis', *The Lancet Infect Dis*, 13(3) (December 20, 2012): 214–22. doi:10.1016/S1473-3099(12)70315-8. PMID: 23260128.

Barry, L., *Images Asia*, personal communication, Chiang Mai, 1996.

Beyrer, C., E. Eiumtrakul, D.D. Celentano, et al., 'Same-sex behavior, sexually transmitted diseases and HIV risks among young northern Thai men', *AIDS*, 9 (1995): 171–6.

Herdt, G., *Same Sex, Different Cultures*, Westview, Boulder, CO, 1997.

Jackson, P., *Male Homosexuality in Thailand*, Global Academic Press, New York, 1989.

Kunawarawak, P., P. Parapunya, C. Natpratan, et al., 'KAP and associated risk factor survey of HIV infection among male commercial sex workers in Chiang Mai, December 1992', presentation at the 11th Annual Health Sciences Meeting, Chiang Mai University, 1993.

Lubis, I., J. Master, M. Bambang, et al., 'AIDS related attitudes and sexual practices of the Jakarta Waria (male transvestites)', *Southeast Asian Journal of Tropical Medicine and Public Health*, 25 (1994): 102–6.

Nanda, S., 'Hijras: an alternative sex and gender role in India', in G. Herdt (ed.), *Third Sex, Third Gender: Beyond Sexual Dimorphism in Culture and History*, Zone Books, New York, 1996, 373–418.

Nopkesorn, T., M. Sweat, S. Kaensing, et al., 'Sexual behaviors for HIV infection in young men in Payao', Research Report No. 6, Program on AIDS, Thai Red Cross Society, 1993.

Patankar, A. (ed.), *The Kamasutra of Vatsyayana*, Hippocrene Books, New York, 1991.

Peltier, A.R., *Pathamamulamuli*, Suriwong Books, Chiang Mai, 1991.

Pradeep, K., M.S. Kumar, Nagarajan, et al., 'Intervention development with men who have sex with men in Madras', 10th International Conference on AIDS, Yokohama, Abstract PD0158, 1994.

Rodrigue, Y., *Nat Pwe: Burma's Supernatural Sub-Culture*, Weatherhill, London, 1995.

Sittitrai, W, T. Brown and C. Sakondhavat, 'Levels of HIV risk behavior and AIDS knowledge in Thai men having sex with men', *AIDS Care*, 5 (1993): 261–71.

Traisupa, A., C. Wongba and D. Taylor, 'AIDS and prevalence of antibody to Human Immunodeficiency Virus (HIV) in high risk groups in Thailand', *Genitourinary Medicine*, 63 (1987): 106–8.

16 *Chaai Chuay Chaai*

Beyrer, C., A. Artenstein, K. Piyada, et al., 'The molecular epidemiology of HIV1 among male commercial sex workers in northern Thailand', *Journal of AIDS and Human Retrovirology*, 15 (1997): 304–7.

de Lind van Wijngaarden, J.W., 'Characteristics, identities, homosexual behavior and condom use among young men in public spaces in urban Chiang Mai, northern Thailand', *NAPAC*, special report, Chiang Mai, 1995.

Guadamuz, T.E., P. Kunawararak, C. Beyrer, et al., 'HIV prevalence, sexual and behavioral correlates among Shan, hill tribe, and Thai male sex workers in Northern Thailand', *AIDS Care*, 16 (April 2010): 1–9.

Kunawararak, P., C. Beyrer, C. Natpratan, et al., 'The epidemiology of HIV and syphilis among male commercial sex workers in northern Thailand', *AIDS*, 9 (1995): 517–21.

Varakitphokatorn, S., 'AIDS risk among tourists: a study of Japanese female tourists in Thailand', technical consultation on information regarding population movements and HIV/AIDS, Chulalongkorn University, Bangkok, 1995.

17 Prisons and prisoners

Amnesty International, 'Myanmar: conditions in prisons and labor camps', *ASA* 16/22/95, September 1995.

Brien, P.M. and A.J. Beck, *HIV in Prisons, 1994*, U.S. Department of Justice, Bureau of Justice Statistics, Publication NCJ-158020, Washington, D.C., 1996.

Choopanya, K., S. Vanichseni, D.C. Des Jarlais, et al., 'Risk factors and HIV seropositivity among injecting drugs users in Bangkok', *AIDS*, 5 (1991): 1509–13.

Correctional Populations in the United States, 1993, U.S. Department of Justice, Bureau of Justice Statistics, Publication NJ-156241, Washington, D.C., 1995.

Gaiter, J. and L.S. Doll, 'Improving HIV/AIDS prevention in prisons is good public health policy', *American Journal of Public Health*, 86 (1996): 1201–3.

Mahon, N., 'New York inmates' HIV risk behaviors: the implications for prevention policy and programs', *American Journal of Public Health*, 86 (1996): 1211–15.

Sprague, L., 'African Americans, HIV, and mass incarceration', *The Lancet*, (14 July, 2016). http://dx.doi.org/10.1016/SO140-6736(16)30830-3.

Walmsley, R., *World Prison Population List* (10th edn), International Centre for Prison Studies and the University of Essex, London, 2013.

Win Naing, O., *Cries from Insein*, All Burma Students Democratic Front, Bangkok, 1996.

Wright, N.H., S. Vanichseni, P. Akarasewi, et al., 'Was the 1988 HIV epidemic among Bangkok's injecting drug users a common source outbreak?', *AIDS*, 8 (1994): 529–32.

18 Activists

Anon., 'The bad neighbor', *Wall Street Journal*, editorial, November 18, 1996.

New Light of Myanmar, 'The people's desire', printed in each daily edition.

19 Drug wars and the war on drugs

Anon., 'Burma's heroin deal', *The Boston Globe*, editorial, November 27, 1996.

Bernstein, D. and L. Kean, 'People of the opiate: Burma's dictatorship of drugs', *The Nation*, December 16, 1996, 11–18.

Beyrer, C., K. Malinowska-Sempruch, A. Kamarulzaman, et al., 'Time to act: a call for comprehensive responses to HIV in people who use drugs', *The Lancet*, 376(9740) (August 14, 2010): 551–63.

Chee Soon Juan, 'Singapore sling', *Dateline Interview*, Australian Broadcasting Service, October 12, 1996.

Csete, J., A. Kamarulzaman, M. Kazatchkine, et al., 'Public health and international drug policy', *The Lancet*, 387(10026) (April 2, 2016): 1427–80. doi:10.1016/S0140-6736(16)00619-X. Review. PMID: 27021149.

Degenhardt, L., B.M. Mathers, A.L. Wirtz, et al., 'What has been achieved in HIV prevention, treatment and care for people who inject drugs, 2010–2012? A review of the six highest burden countries', *Int J Drug Policy*, (September 4, 2013). doi:10.1016/j.drugpo.2013.08.004.

McCoy, A.W, C.B. Reed and C.P. Adams, *The Politics of Heroin in Southeast Asia*, Harper & Row, Singapore, 1972.

Parliament of the Commonwealth of Australia, *A Report on Human Rights and the Lack of Progress Towards Democracy in Burma (Myanmar): The Drug Trade*, Joint Standing Committee of Foreign Affairs, Defense and Trade, Canberra, 1995.

Razak, M.H., J. Jittiwutikarn, V. Suriyanon, et al., 'HIV prevalence and risks among injection and non-injection drug users in northern Thailand: need for comprehensive HIV prevention programs', *J AIDS*, 33(2) (2003): 259–66.

Whitman, W., *Specimen Days*, edited by Mark Van Doren, Viking Press, New York, 1945.

20 Brethren

Aengus Carroll, International Lesbian, Gay, Bisexual, Trans and Intersex Association (ILGA), *State Sponsored Homophobia*, ILGA Annual Report, May 2016.

Baral, S., F. Sifakis, F. Cleghorn, et al., 'Elevated risk for HIV infection among men who have sex with men in low and middle income countries 2000–2006: results of a meta-analysis', *PLoS Med*, 4(12) (December 2007): e339.

Beyrer, C., 'Pushback: the current wave of anti-homosexuality laws and impacts on health', *PLoS Med*, 11(6) (June 24, 2014): e1001658.

Beyrer, C., S.D. Baral, C. Collins, et al., 'The global response to HIV in men who have sex with men', *The Lancet*, 388(10040) (July 9, 2016): 198–206. doi:10.1016/S0140-6736(16)30781-4.

Beyrer, C., S.D. Baral, F. van Griensven, et al., 'Global epidemiology of HIV infection in men who have sex with men', *The Lancet*, 380(9839) (July 28, 2012): 367–77. PMID: 22819660.

Beyrer, C., S.D. Baral, D. Walker, et al., 'The expanding epidemics of HIV-1 among men who have sex with men in low and middle income countries: diversity and consistency', *Epidemiol Rev*, 32(1) (April 2010): 137–51.

Beyrer, C., P.S. Sullivan, J. Sanchez, et al., 'A call to action for comprehensive HIV services for men who have sex with men', *The Lancet*, 380(9839) (July 28, 2012): 424–38. PMID: 22819663.

Mayer, K.H., D.P. Wheeler, L.G. Bekker, et al., 'Overcoming biological, behavioral, and structural vulnerabilities: new directions in research to decrease HIV transmission in men who have sex with men', *J AIDS*, 63 (Suppl. 2) (July 2013): S161–7. doi:10.1097/QAI.0b013e318298700e. PMID: 23764630.

Trapence, G., C. Collins, S. Avrett, et al., 'From personal survival to public health: community leadership by men who have sex with men in the response to HIV', *The Lancet*, 380(9839) (July 28, 1012): 400–410. PMID: 22819662.

21 Medical ethics, human rights, Asian values

Beyrer, C., 'Responding to epidemic disease threats in Burma and lessons for China: why good governance matters', in S.R. Quah (ed.), *Crisis Preparedness: Asia and the Global Governance of Epidemics*. The Walter H. Shorenstein Asia-Pacific Research Center, Stanford, CA, 2007, 47–62.

Cohen, R. and L.S. Wiseberg, *Double Jeopardy: Threat to Life and Human Rights. Discrimination against Persons with AIDS*, Human Rights Internet, Harvard Law School, Cambridge, MA, 1990.

Farmer, P., *AIDS and Accusation: Haiti and the Geography of Blame*, University of California Press, Berkeley, CA, 1992.

Lintner, B. and H.N. Lintner, 'Blind in Rangoon: AIDS epidemic rages, but the junta says no to NGOs', *Far Eastern Economic Review*, August 1, 1991, 21.

MacKinnon, C., 'Crimes of war, crimes of peace', in S. Shute and S. Hurley (eds), *On Human Rights, The Oxford Amnesty Lectures 1993*, Basic Books, New York, 1993, 83–109.

Panos Institute, *The 3rd Epidemic: Repercussions of the Fear of AIDS*, The Panos Institute, London, 1990.

22 The proper study of mankind

Beyrer, C. 'The proper study of mankind', *The Lancet*, 386(10005) (October 31, 2015): 1724–5. doi:10.1016/S0140-6736(15)61217-X. PMID: 26545422.

Beyrer, C., J.C. Villar, V. Suwanvanichkij, et al., 'Neglected diseases, civil conflicts and the right to health', *The Lancet*, 370(9587) (August 2007): 619–27.

Orbinski, J., C. Beyrer, S. Singh, et al., 'Violations of human rights: health practitioners as witnesses', *The Lancet*, 370(9588) (August 2007): 698–704.

Shantideva, 'A guide to the Bodhisattva's way of life', translated by S. Batchelor, Library of Tibetan Works and Archives, Dharamsala, 1979.

Tenzin Gyatso HH, The 14th Dalai Lama, *The Mind's Own Physician: A Dialogue with the Dalai Lama on the Healing Power of Meditation*, edited by J. Kabat-Zinn and R.J. Davidson, New Harbinger, Oakland, CA, 2011.

Tenzin Gyatso HH, The 14th Dalai Lama, *Kindness, Clarity, and Insight*, translated by J. Hopkins, Snow Lion, Boston, MA, 2012.

Williams, W.C. *The Autobiography of William Carlos Williams*, New Directions, San Francisco, CA, 1967.

INDEX